D0971120

healing WORDS *for*
HEALING people

healing **WORDS** *for* **HEALING** people

PRAYERS AND MEDITATIONS FOR PARISH NURSES AND OTHER HEALTH PROFESSIONALS

DEBORAH L. PATTERSON

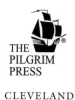

THE
PILGRIM
PRESS

CLEVELAND

DEDICATION

To the nurses, doctors,
chaplains, and parish clergy who have lived before
and live today as God's healers
and to those all dear ones with whom I live and work,
who bring healing and hope to me.

The Pilgrim Press, 700 Prospect Avenue, Cleveland, Ohio 44115-1100
thepilgrimpress.com
© 2005 by Deborah L. Patterson

Biblical quotations are primarily from the New Revised Standard Version of the Bible. © 1989 by the Division of Christian Education of the National Council of the Churches of Christ in the U.S.A., and are used by permission.

10 09 08 07 06 05   5 4 3 2 1

Library of Congress Cataloging-in-Publication Data

Patterson, Deborah L., 1956 -
    Healing words for healing people: prayers and meditations for parish nurses and other health professionals/Deborah Patterson.
        p. cm.
    Includes bibliographical references.
    ISBN 0-8298-1673-9 (paper : alk. paper)
    1. Parish nursing — Prayer-books and devotions — English. 2. Medical personnel — Prayer-books and devotions — English. I. Title.

BV4596.N8P38 2005
242'.68—dc22

                                                            2005051489

CONTENTS

preface...9

meditations

prayers

preface

Once upon a time, clergy and nurses and doctors worked together. There was not a cavernous divide between science and theology. Ministers believed in good science, and doctors and nurses believed in good theology.

Once upon a time, there wasn't as much to know about medicine and nursing as there is today. When many church-related hospitals were being founded in the nineteenth century, there were no antibiotics, few anesthetics, and only rudimentary surgical instruments and diagnostic equipment. Prayer was an important tool for the patient and often for the doctor as well. Nobody expected a heart transplant. In those days, the clergy could do nearly as much for the person with heart disease as the doctor or nurse. Those days are over.

Once upon a time, the pursuit of theology involved a serious course of study for academics, who learned the ancient languages in which sacred texts were written and were familiar with the sociohistoric settings in which their faiths were grounded. Many took public stands on important social issues and were involved in the founding and running of hospitals, among other social institutions. Theologians attempting to bring new theological insights to social issues today are branded as infidels. Few theologians are found among upper echelons of healthcare organizations; they have become irrelevant.

In America, we routinely expect the medical profession to "make us well." We expect the nursing staff to "take care of us." We see clergy occasionally, if someone is getting married or needs burial (a "failure" of medical science). The clergy comprise the "clean-up squad."

We also see doctors and nurses suffering from stress, addictions, and burnout at unprecedented rates. We see large numbers of clergy who are depressed. We are all too often divorced from our own wholeness — we can do a great deal for others, but we are so in need of care ourselves!

This book is written on the premise that clergy, doctors, and nurses are all needed in the search for human wholeness. They have a lot in common. All those for whom they tend need the care of body, mind, and soul. Clergy, doctors, and nurses need self-care of their own bodies, minds, and souls. Parish nurses, holistic health nurses, growing numbers of other nurses, physicians, and clergy are joining this search for integration between spirituality and health. This book is for them.

My purpose in collecting the prayers and meditations in this book is to remind us that we are not alone. They speak of God's never-ending love for us all, no matter what our circumstances or physical condition. They speak of the love of others who hold us in prayer so we may know that we are not alone. They speak of hope and promise and courage.

My prayer this day is that these prayers and meditations may be a source of healing and peace for you and those with whom you minister, as one of God's healers, in a world so much in need of the gifts that you have to share.

I would like to add a word of thanks to those who have shared their gifts with me. Helen Westberg and her children, especially John Westberg and Jill Westberg McNamara, are a source of great inspiration and blessing as they continue the legacy of Helen's husband, the Rev. Dr. Granger Westberg. Rev. Westberg was the impetus behind many conversations between clergy and health professionals, and the founder of parish nursing. Thanks also to parish nurse educators, coordinators, and parish nurses, whose cutting-edge work on the integration of faith and health both blesses and inspires. In my capacity as the executive director of the International Parish Nurse Resource Center, it is my privilege to work with many of these pioneering souls on a daily basis.

Thanks also to those who have read this manuscript and shared their wisdom. I am grateful to my friend and colleague, Rev. Jerry W. Paul, the president and CEO of the Deaconess Foundation, who has encouraged my work and provided helpful feedback in myriad ways over the last ten years. Norella Huggins, a board member of Deaconess for over fifteen years, provided many healing words to this manuscript, as did Dee Mehl Ban, a wonderful artist with music and words. I am grateful to several other coworkers, colleagues, and friends for their help and suggestions, including Dr. Nesa Joseph, Dr. David Ban, Dr. Lewis Wall, Rev. Katherine Hawker, Laura Rein, Rev. Dr. Allen Mueller, Alvyne Rethemeyer, Barbara Wehling, Maureen Daniels, and Sister Marian Cowan. I would like to give a special word of thanks to Kim Sadler, Editorial Director at The Pilgrim Press, for her helpful style of encouragement and grace, to Aimee Jahnsohn and Janice Brown, also at The Pilgrim Press, and to Linda Cuckovich for her skilled and gracious copyediting. And I am forever grateful to my husband, Steve, and my children Sophia and John, for their boundless love.

Finally, I offer thanks to those professionals in the many hospitals, clinics, nursing homes, and churches who get up each day and go to work, faithful to their call to care for and about others. Their healing words and work continue to call forth hope for so many.

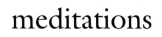

meditations

1

Placing Your Prayer Order

The Spirit helps us in our weakness, for we do not know how to pray as we ought, but that very Spirit intercedes for us with sighs too deep for words.
(Romans 8:26)

"Faith and health" have become fashionable commodities these days. In *Healing Words,* his best-seller on prayer, Larry Dossey, M.D., a physician who takes both spirituality and medical science very seriously, undertook the daunting task of reviewing "over one hundred experiments exhibiting the criteria of 'good science,' many conducted under stringent laboratory conditions, over half of which showed that prayer brings about significant changes in a variety of living beings."[1] His findings raise the question, however: What about that other half?

Prayer is not like placing an order at a fast-food drive-through. One can't pull up to the speaker, yell, "Heal Aunt Millie, please," and pull around to the window to pick her up doing cartwheels out of the ICU.

Certainly we in health care and in religious circles have prayed for others who have miraculously recovered from illness. We have all prayed for others who, despite our efforts, have tragically died. Many have prayed for healing from chronic diseases and pain that just won't go away. Does this mean that God only answers some prayers? What is the effectiveness of prayer, of these healing words? The problem with "prayer experiments" is that they are inherently flawed by their very nature, or, more accurately, by the nature of God. The subjects — in one instance mice who had been purposely cut or injected with malaria — were separated into "prayed-for" and "not-prayed-for" groups. But would God, being loving and just, not care equally about all these little creatures? Would not God perhaps care even more for the ones who had no one to pray for their wounded bodies? What sort of God would care only for those who are the object of our prayers and not for the lost and lonely without a "prayer team" in their corner? Would such a God be worthy of our prayers and our worship? Whatever is going on in such experiments, I suspect it has very little to do with God.

The very fact that human beings conceive of and conduct prayer experiments does tell us something profound about the nature of humankind, however. Prayer experiments are performed to study another avenue of healing, to leave no stone unturned in the search for wholeness and the alleviation of suffering. God is in relationship with human beings who care deeply about the welfare of others — enough to dedicate energy and time, in fact, entire careers to bring healing resources to others.

Robert Frost railed against building false divisions and walls in the world in his famous poem, "Mending Wall."[2] Even as he repaired the wall with his neighbor he noticed that we are, with nature, beings who long for the world to be whole, not divided. We are seeking connection and wellness, what is called "spirituality and health" these days. We are seeking relation to the other — other people, other creatures, and "the other" as glimpsed through our experiences of the transcendent reality known to us in many names, often called God.

The deep, abiding value of prayer, I believe, is that it reminds us of our connection to God and to others. Dossey himself illustrates this well when he speaks of a man dying from lung cancer:

> The day before his death, I sat at his bedside with his wife and children. He knew he had little time left and he chose his words carefully, speaking in a hoarse whisper. Although not a religious person, he revealed to us that recently he had begun to pray frequently.
>
> "What do you pray for?" I asked.
>
> "I don't pray for anything," he responded. "How would I know what to ask for?" This was surprising. Surely this

dying man could think of some request.

"If prayer is not for asking, what is it *for?*" I pushed him.

"It isn't *for* anything," he said thoughtfully. "It reminds me that I am not alone."[3]

It is hard to pray. Sometimes uttering a word of prayer is the hardest thing on earth. Sometimes we are stubborn, stiff-necked, independent, "do-it-yourself" people. We don't believe that God will hear. We don't believe that anyone will hear. We don't believe that anyone will care, even if they do hear. We don't believe that anyone will answer. And we don't believe that anything will change.

It is easy to pray. One word is enough: "Help!" "God!" "Allah!" "Jesus!" "Savior!" Sometimes we find a prayer we know well can help us more than anything — the Lord's Prayer, the Hail Mary, the Shemah. Sometimes the prayers pour out of us like water, like blood.

There is no right way to pray. There are many paths. Pray on your knees, on your back, on your feet. Pray as you wake, or before you go to sleep. Pray in thanksgiving before you eat, or for guidance before you begin your work. Jesus said, "Pray constantly."

Among the most heart-rending things I hear in my work are stories of people who are experiencing great emotional or physical pain, but who feel they *can't* pray because they don't know how. The apostle Paul says, "The Spirit helps us in our weakness, for we do not know how to pray as we ought, but that very Spirit intercedes for us with sighs too deep for words" (Romans 8:26). Just breathe. Just talk. Just listen. Just think about God, love, hope, compassion, healing, connection. Listen for the Spirit.

Healers are very susceptible to burnout. Healers often leave prayer to the edges of their lives because they are so very busy. They work with so many people, many of whom have so many needs. A healer's work is never done. Prayer is often left to the experts — to the chaplains, or even better, to really outstanding pray-ers, like Billy Graham or someone who has written famous books on prayer, like George Buttrick.

Can you breathe? Can you think? Can you talk? If you can do any of these things, you can pray. You don't have to pray. But you can. You don't have to listen for the still, small words of God for your life. But you can. You don't have to pray for others. But you can. And in praying you will be blessed. Perhaps those for whom you pray will be blessed because you will be refreshed as you come to work with them, and they will be refreshed by knowing that someone cares enough about them to lift them up into the light of the presence of the transcendent.

The way God's love breaks into pain and suffering and brings transformation and hope can be surprising. Healers want interventions that work. What if prayer works in a way that we can't measure or understand? What if healing happens that we never see — healing that looks far different from that for which we were praying? It's a great big universe out there. We don't know everything yet!

Healing words should be words that heal. They should be words of forgiveness, of hope, of compassion. Healing words should be words that assure the patient, the patient's family, and us that we are never alone. Healing words should help patients take courage and strength in the thought that healers will stand with them, no matter what. Healing words should assure us that there is nowhere we can be or go beyond the reach of God's abiding love.

God loves us whether we pray or not. Always. No matter what. And prayer might help us believe it. Amen.

2

The Kindness of Strangers

Finally, beloved, whatever is true, whatever is honorable, whatever is just, whatever is pure, whatever is pleasing, whatever is commendable, if there is any excellence and if there is anything worthy of praise, think about these things. (Philippians 4:8)

Recently I had the opportunity to visit the Holocaust Museum in Washington, D.C. As one enters the main exhibit, there are several boxes labeled "male" and "female" on a small table. Inside the boxes are "passports" for the visitors. Each passport tells the story of someone who went through the Holocaust. The museum has four floors corresponding to the passage of time during the 1930s and 1940s. One page of the passport is to be turned at the end of each floor.

The museum itself defies description. There are photographs of children, women, and men who died, film clips from newscasts of the day, maps of towns in which Gestapo prisons and work camps were located. There are pictures of victims undergoing "medical experimentation" authorized by the Nazis. One room is simply a wooden walkway, surrounded by a musty landscape of slowly decaying leather shoes of every size, left to bear witness to the dead. Altogether, over six million people were murdered in the Holocaust, among them 200,000 Romani (Gypsies), 10,000 homosexual men and women, many dissidents, including Rev. Dietrich Bonhoeffer, and two out of every three European Jews.

The passport that was chosen for me told the story of a Jewish woman from Lvov, Poland (near the town in which my grandmother was born), who survived through the kindness of strangers. One man helped her get false identity papers. Another person helped her find a job. Later she escaped to Canada, where she married another Holocaust survivor. They now live in the United States.

Walking through the museum, one feels many things. One wonders, "How could this happen? Could this happen to me? Could I do such a thing to others? Would I have helped those who were so desperate?" The awful thing about these questions is that we know that each human being is capable of terrible indifference and even cruelty.

It has been several decades since the Holocaust, but we must not forget what can happen to the human spirit in times of great pressure. War is still a constant presence in our world.

Our struggle with the choice between indifference and compassion is a daily one. Make no mistake, compassion must include objectivity and boundaries in order for care to be professional. But indifference can be deadly. Healers are under extreme stress right now because they see so many people who are falling through the cracks, so many people who need care. Every person who becomes ill and comes into the care of health-care professionals is dependent upon the kindness of strangers. No one can give themselves surgery or radiation treatment. People who are looking to health professionals for care depend on compassion to help them through. Those who are terminally ill depend on the kindness of strangers to help them in their dying. And healers are those strangers who make a place for kindness and compassion.

The apostle Paul, a Jewish man writing to some Greek strangers in the church at Phillipi, writes, "Finally, brothers and sisters, whatever is true, whatever is honorable, whatever is just, whatever is pure, whatever is lovely, whatever is gracious, if there is any excellence, if there is anything worthy of praise, think about these things. What you have learned and received and seen in me, do; and the God of peace will be with you" (Philippians 4:8-9).

We are all strangers on this earth, and yet we are all connected, one to the other, by the God who has called forth each one who lives. May the God of peace be with you, as you seek what is true and honorable, as you strive for justice and compassion.

Shalom.

3

All Good Things

Give us this day our daily bread, and forgive us our debts, as we also have
forgiven our debtors. And do not bring us into the time of trial, but rescue us
from the evil one.
Matthew 6:11-13

Awhile back, in the midst of a spate of gloomy rain, I walked over to the
St. Louis Art Museum for a few minutes after work at the hospital.
Somehow, looking at beautiful things from ages past gives us the sense of
being part of something larger than ourselves, part of a grand adventure
known as life, with all of its creativity and joy, mundane worries and fiery
passions, coursing through the centuries.

I poked my head into an exhibit called "Splendor of the Pharaohs," where
a stony face caught my eye. It was a faintly green statue of the god Osiris,
with his arms folded in majestic dignity. Osiris was the Egyptian god associated
with new vegetation and was considered a renewer of all life. This particular
figure, about 2,700 years old, had been commissioned by a "royal acquain-
tance" named Ptahirdis. He had the statue made with a prayer to Osiris on
the back. The inscription says, "May you give me bread, beer, and all good
things. May you rescue me from all things evil. May you give me power."

It is somehow heartwarming to know that someone 2,700 years ago
was worried about the same kind of things we worry about. "Give us our
daily bread," we pray. "Deliver us from evil. Thine is the power." Our
understanding of God has certainly changed since the days of the Pharaohs,
but we still long for connection to a caring presence beyond ourselves.
We still worry about feeding our families, about keeping them safe, about

finding meaning and purpose in our lives, and having the power to make a difference.

The minister and theologian Reinhold Niebuhr once put this prayer another way. Speaking at a small church in Heath, Massachusetts, during the Great Depression in 1934, he prayed, "O God, give us serenity to accept what cannot be changed, courage to change what should be changed, and wisdom to distinguish the one from the other."[1] This prayer has come to be known as "The Serenity Prayer," and the words generally changed to "give me" from "give us." However, Niebuhr had a different intent behind this prayer that was not simply personal piety. According to biographer June Bingham in *The Courage to Change*, his prayer should more aptly be entitled "The Courage Prayer."[2] For Niebuhr, finding courage to change the things we should was the most important part of his petitions to God and to humankind and a religious person's most important task. He spoke out for peace and justice all the days of his life, first as a pastor in Detroit during Henry Ford's days, and later as a professor at Union Seminary in New York City during World War II. Even though he always thought of himself as rather shy, he somehow found the courage to speak out to improve the lives of others. He couldn't change the stroke that left him unable to speak late in his life, but his courage and wisdom continue to speak to us today.

In health care we have the privilege of walking with people at times in their lives when they are vulnerable and often afraid. We are entrusted with the care of human lives and the hopes and dreams of which they are built. This is a calling that requires great courage. Where does such courage come from? We all, like Ptahirdis and Niebuhr, long for God to walk with us, to help us through the trials and tribulations we face. These are timeless concerns. The apostle Paul spoke words of courage when he said: "For I am sure that neither death, nor life, nor angels, nor principalities, nor things present, nor things to come, nor powers, nor height, nor depth, nor anything else in all creation will be able to separate us from the love of God in Christ Jesus our Lord" (Romans 8:38).

So enjoy the day in which you find yourself. Be at peace as you care for those who come to you. Know that you are not alone — that God cares for them and for you. Have courage, serenity, and wisdom, and may you have bread, beer (or a heart-healthy nonalcoholic beverage), and all good things.

4

The Healing Power of Doing Good

Strive first for the kingdom of God and his righteousness, and all these things will be given to you as well.
Matthew 6:33

A few years ago, my husband and I were awakened in the middle of the night, pulled from a deep sleep by the strong smell of smoke. It smelled like burning wires, and we feared an electrical fire in the walls. Some of you may know how utterly terrifying that smell is in the middle of the night. We ran downstairs and tried to locate the source of the smoke. It seemed to be strongest in the kitchen, but there were no flames. We dialed 911.

As soon as I got off the phone with the dispatcher, I turned around. There, heating on the stove, was our copper-bottomed teakettle. Or more accurately, our formerly copper-bottomed tea kettle, left by mistake on the lit burner for hours, the obvious source of the fumes.

Luckily, we were able to cancel the 911 call before the trucks left the station. But what a profoundly grateful feeling it gave us to know they were there, to know that people were at the firehouse, day and night, to try to help where needed. We turned off the scorched kettle and breathed a sigh of relief. We went back to bed very thankful indeed.

Most of us have a great deal to be thankful for. We know how tenuous life is, how fleeting, how fragile. Who has not felt that fragility in the middle of the night? Who has not lifted prayers for worries that have come near to us? Perhaps it was worry for our safety. Perhaps it was worry about a loved one, worry about health, worry about work. The cares of the world touch us all, young and old, rich and poor.

It was to address those very real worries that a group of people in Miami started a volunteer program. The program invited senior citizens to volunteer to help others in need. Each volunteer received credit for work performed, and that credit later could be cashed in, if ever he/she was in need of help. Those in the program would not need to worry that they would be left alone. What the organizers of the program discovered, however, was rather startling. After several years of the program, nearly 90,000 credits had been earned for volunteer hours given. Yet only 1 percent of those credits had ever been used. The organizers of the program found that those people who volunteered to help had improved health, and very few of them needed to cash in their credits.

Allen Luks, in his book, *The Healing Power of Doing Good*, discusses this phenomenon. He documents many studies that show that people who volunteer to help others become healthier and happier themselves. Helping out of obligation generally does not bring these benefits. Rather, the "healing power of doing good" is brought through the joy of helping a stranger, of touching the life of a person you would not have otherwise known, from whom you could have easily walked away. It is the pleasure of seeing a life changed, a small difference made. It is the benefit of seeking first the realm of God, and God's righteousness and justice.

Luks tells the story of a woman named Lynn, who comforted babies who had been born addicted to crack. As she rocked and cooed to the children, she found her chronic back pain abating.[1] He writes also of Randee, whose fiancée was killed before her eyes in a car accident. Years later she became a volunteer for a hospice program and healed her own heart.[2] Perhaps the most dramatic story he tells, though, is the story of a small town in France.

Le Chambon-sur-Lignon is a little village nestled in a mountain valley in the Haute-Loire region of southern France. Some of the people who live there are Huguenots (French Protestants); others are Catholic. Their ancestors had known great persecution and trauma. It would be easy for these people to shut out the world.

But the world came to their doorsteps in the middle of the night during World War II. It came in the form of a woman, a woman who was German and Jewish. She came to the door of Magna Trocme, wife of the Huguenot minister. When Magna was asked by the woman for shelter and a hiding place, she did not hesitate. "Come in," she said.

The Church Council voted to stand behind their pastor and his wife. Over the next few years, the entire town, Protestant and Catholic, agreed to help. Jewish children slept in barns and stables of farms all around town. One village boy was in charge of a system to warn the children if they needed to stay hidden. If the shutters of his room were open, they could join the others at school. If his shutters were closed, the children were to hurry back into hiding.

Not one refugee from that town was ever turned in. Over five thousand Jews were rescued there. That was a number equal to the entire population of Le Chambon-sur-Lignon.

When movie director Paul Sauvage later visited the town to ask them why they did what they did, the residents shrugged their shoulders. They said, simply, "It was the right thing to do."[3]

"Strive first for the realm of God, and God's righteousness, and all these things will be given to you as well" (Matthew 6:33). This remarkable village responded to the call to seek first God's righteousness. It is the same call that beckons to us in our world today.

The horror of Nazi Germany is over, but there is still pain in our towns and cities. We are called to choose the path that brings life. When Le Chambon-sur-Lignon responded to the needs of German Jews who arrived on their doorsteps, the pain of deep, historic Protestant-Catholic divisions began to heal, as the town worked together to tend others whose lives depended on their unified response.

We are not alone. There are people who will help us in the middle of the night. Firefighters, police officers, ambulance drivers, and healers stand ready in almost every town and village of this country. Many other parts of the world are not so fortunate, but God has not forgotten them. Perhaps God is calling you to serve them. We know that the God of all creation is the God who is by our side, who is calling, who is leading us to journeys of transformation.

We are not alone. There are neighbors and strangers who need our help.

When we reach out to others, we are richly blessed by the God who cares for us all.

So, in the middle of the night, in the middle of your trials, in the middle of your joys, remember. Remember that you are not alone. We are not alone. We are called to care for others, as they are called to care for their neighbors. Our smallest acts of kindness are blessed by the God of righteousness and justice. Le Chambon-sur-Lignon could not save all the Jews, Gypsies, homosexuals, epileptics, developmentally delayed and mentally retarded individuals who were targeted for death by Hitler and his cronies. But Magna saved the woman who came to her door. Lynn couldn't hold every baby who was born addicted to cocaine. But the ones she held were comforted. Randee couldn't sit with every dying person. But the lives she touched changed her forever. We as individuals, as church members, as medical, nursing, chaplaincy, or other staff at hospitals, cannot change the world, but we can change neighborhoods. We can change communities.

In the middle of our giving, we are blessed. In the middle of the night, that blessing sustains us. So have no fear! May you continue to be a blessing and be blessed by the God who made us all.

Amen and amen.

5

When Did We Welcome You?

Truly, I tell you, just as you did it to one of the least of these who are members of my family, you did it to me.
Matthew 25:40

In her book, *Everyday Sacred,* Sue Bender writes about a man named Martin, who works in the busy Berkeley café she visits early each morning. As he serves each person in line, Martin takes one extra moment to form, with a spoon, a smile in the foam of each cappuccino. He doesn't have to do this. It isn't a "gimmick" at the café or an empty act like the hollow "have a nice day" one hears too often. It seems hokey, yet the thought of someone drawing a smile in one's coffee can't help but make me smile. It would get me off to a good start. Sue Bender says of the man, "Martin is shy, and in this situation I am also shy. We hardly talk, but his act of generosity blesses my day."[1]

One sees this often in the healing professions. People who come to these professions often are drawn from something inside of them. We all need a sense of purpose, of participating in something larger than ourselves, of contributing to a greater good. Martin expresses his philosophy by stating, "Work is very important for me…. I think people appreciate what I have done…. I want something *inside,* more than money or material things."[2]

The organization for which I work, "Deaconess Parish Nurse Ministries," was started at the Deaconess Hospital in St. Louis. The root from which the English word "deaconess" comes from is the Greek word "diakonia" and means "table-service." People in the early church were called to serve others in the community by meeting the needs of the poor, orphans, widows, and foreigners, both in body and soul. It sprang from a feeling of gratitude for what God had done for them. That gratitude prompted people in the church to begin hospitals, and many hospitals bear names like "Deaconess" or "St. John's" even today. The Sisters of Charity of the Incarnate Word began their work in San Antonio, Texas, in 1869 in response to a call for help from Bishop Claude Marie Dubuis, who stated, "Our Lord Jesus Christ, suffering in the persons of a multitude of the sick and infirm of every kind, seeks relief at your hands."[3] They knew they were serving God in the people they served.

The gospel writer Matthew put it this way: "'Lord, when did we see you hungry and feed you, or thirsty and give you something to drink? And when did we see you a stranger and welcome you, or naked and clothe you? And when did we see you sick or in prison and visit you?' And Jesus will answer them, 'Truly, I say to you, as you did it to one of the least of these my brothers and sisters, you did it to me'" (Matthew 25:37-40).

I am sure that there are as many reasons for working in health care or the ministry as there are people in these fields. We are surrounded by a great cloud of witnesses — people who have gone before and shared their gifts and talents generously with those in need of care. And we are surrounded by others here and now who inspire us with excellence and compassion each day. Hang in there, my friends. As you drink smiling coffee (or serious Diet Coke) and as you go through your day touching others in their intimate need, may God bless your work and your soul.

Amen.

6

All Will Be Well

I praise you, for I am fearfully and wonderfully made. Wonderful are your works; that I know very well.
Psalm 139:14

My father is a grass fanatic. He and my mother live on a farm in Alberta, Canada, where the summer sun rises early and lingers long into the evening. Consequently, the grass grows quickly, which my dad takes as a personal challenge. He wants a perfect lawn for the entire six weeks when it doesn't snow.

Dad goes out every couple of days on the riding mower to mow down the lane and around the farm buildings. Then he chooses a push mower from his arsenal of equipment in the shed and cuts the grass surrounding the houses (theirs and the house that was my grandma's). Finally, he completes the conquest with a weed whacker, an edge trimmer, and nostril tweezers.

My family and I fly up there from St. Louis each summer to visit. One summer before making our annual pilgrimage north we took a short vacation at an ecumenical retreat center called Ring Lake Ranch near Dubois, Wyoming. This was a place that would have driven my dad crazy. Ring Lake Ranch's philosophy is, "Do not interfere with nature." The grounds were covered with sagebrush and prairie weeds, rocks, and decaying scrub trees. It was an absolutely glorious mess, which nature most often is when left to its own devices. Nature's beautiful messiness violates our sense of order and defies our need to control things.

We are constantly working with the forces of nature as healers. Birth, growth, disease, healing, aging, and death are all part of this glorious mess we know as life. We try to control nature as much as possible, but we recognize that there is something greater than ourselves at work.

From the front window of our cabin at the ranch we had a magnificent view of the Absoroka mountain range and Ring Lake. However, smack-dab in the middle of that picture window was a dead tree, screaming its demise to a world filled with beauty and health. My reaction (the one I learned mastering the mower with training wheels) was to pull it out, get rid of it, make certain that everything stayed green, fully alive, and in its proper place.

Yet perhaps it is precisely when we fully experience the presence of one who is dying that we can see most clearly the beauty of life. We know that each day is precious, a gift from God. We know that ultimately we all will die. We know that there is nothing greater than to have lived, and loved, and to have done something meaningful. Those who linger near death testify that there is great value in life, even in its closing days, which must be treasured.

We may not know what to say to those who are dying when there is nothing more that we can do to "cure" them, but the dying may have something of importance to say to us. Perhaps they may tell us that they are ready to embrace their passage through death. Perhaps their journey may remind us to live each day to the fullest, knowing that we all will die. Perhaps their message would resemble that of Julian of Norwich (a religious woman who lived in the late-fourteenth and early-fifteenth centuries) who said, "All will be well." Or they might simply like the opportunity to bid us farewell.

What can we say to them as we face our own mortality? We can say, "We have done all we could." We need to be honest with each person. We can say, "We suggest you consider hospice." There, the dying receives compassionate care in their own homes, surrounded by their friends and family. We can say, "We care about you." We can say, "We will pray for you." And we might also take the opportunity to thank them and to say, "Good-bye."

When we are afraid of the dying, something within ourselves dies. We lose touch with the reality of our own mortality and its inestimable contribution to the value of our human lives. But when we have the courage to walk with them through their hardest journey, we gain a deeper understanding of the mystery of life.

A great new interest in spirituality is occurring these days, and healers are playing a part in this. As science unravels more of the mysteries of the human body and the processes of living and dying, we find we grow closer to Mystery. We are fearfully and wonderfully made. And God is part of it all.

So enjoy God's blessings as you revel in the glorious mess that life is! Enjoy these precious days. All will be well.

Amen.

7

When to Go Home

For in six days the Lord made heaven and earth, the sea, and all that is in them, but rested the seventh day.
Exodus 20:11a

Marian Wright Edelman, the founder and president of the Children's Defense Fund, writes the following prayer in her book, *Guide My Feet:* "Lord, help me to sort out what I should do first, second, and third today and to not try to do everything at once and nothing well. Give me the wisdom to delegate what I can and to order the things I can't delegate, to say no when I need to, and the sense to know when to go home."[1]

When I read this prayer, I laughed out loud and thought, "Has this woman been looking in on my life? Has she been sticking her head around the corner when I haven't been watching?"

Sometimes it seems we are, in this twenty-first-century world, on overload. So many things to do, and so little time. So many needs. So many sick people, so many poor people, so many hungry people, so many lonely people. There is drug addiction in the world, there is violence in the world, there are wars in the world. We know we are called to make a difference, but how, in God's name, can one person make a dent?

Actually, one person can't change the world. But one person can change. And that one person can share the love she/he has experienced in that change with somebody else. And then that person might change. Soon that second person may be sharing compassion with another, and yet a third person could be changed. We seldom know the end result of our work.

I have heard many stories from people whose lives have been touched by others. One woman told me about a kindly nurse who helped her at the end of a difficult pregnancy. Another talked about the marvelous care his dying wife received from hospice. Someone else told about the support staff in the ICU when her close friend was there. A middle-aged man spoke gratefully about a doctor who prayed with him and treated him compassionately and well when he faced a life-threatening diagnosis. They didn't tell the people who helped them, but they told somebody. *Their* lives were changed.

None of us is alone in our healing work. Together, we can make a tremendous difference if each of us stays grounded in reality and perspective. We need to stay connected to the others who are providing care — to others who are working to make a difference. We need to stay connected to those in our homes and lives who support *us* and give *us* love. And most of all, we need to stay connected to the source of all love — God.

Finally, we need one more thing: to know when to go home. Take care of yourselves — you are precious.

Amen.

8

Enough Trouble for Today

So do not worry about tomorrow, for tomorrow will bring worries of its own.
Today's trouble is enough for today.
Matthew 6:34

The worst part of my job is working with people. If I could have just one day at work where I didn't have to answer the telephone, didn't have to go to a meeting, didn't have to talk to anybody, I could get all caught up with my paperwork, clean up my computer files, sort through the stuff on my desk, and finally get to all those journals I have been wanting to read. That would be sublime and my life would be fulfilled. I could die in peace.

The best part of my job is working with people. Every day my life is touched and changed by the lives of others around me. I see people accomplishing incredible things in their work. I see caregivers standing over the bedsides of patients, coaching them on to health. I see students learning new things and growing in their competence each day. I see courage in people's personal lives as they struggle with challenges they never believed would be possible to overcome. This is a blessing to me, and I hope I don't die for a long time. I want to see what other things these amazing people will do.

Come to work. Go home. Come to work. Go home. Pretty much the same every day. Yet between the spaces of these sentences are the stories of people's lives. Babies. Heart attacks. New cars. Car accidents. Kindergarten. Influenza. Every story just a little different, the spin on every life just a little varied. One never knows from one day to the next what is around the corner.

Rabbi Lawrence Kushner, in his book *Invisible Lines of Connection: Sacred Stories of the Ordinary,* talks about a moment in his life when he thought he might have a brain tumor, and was waiting for the results of a CT scan. He writes,

> I felt what I can only call "a trembling deep inside me." And I remember thinking: So this is how it happens. One day, I'm well. Then, suddenly, and almost gracefully, I'm in possession of an all-consuming new piece of information: the probable cause of my imminent death. One minute I'm preoccupied by a thousand daily tasks. And the next, it's as if some hand from out of nowhere had swept everything off the game board and onto the floor and replaced all my affairs with a medical diagnosis.[1]

The people healers see are often frightened and brave. The people who care for the sick are brave, and are facing their own fears. We have no guarantees, only each other. And we have God.

Remembering this helps me put the meetings and all the other job demands back into perspective. People — God's people — make this work worthwhile.

There is a wonderful saying near the end of what is known as the "Sermon on the Mount." Jesus says, "Do not worry about tomorrow, for tomorrow will have worries of its own. Today's trouble is enough for today" (Matthew 6:34). Amen!

Tomorrow will have worries — we never know what is around the corner. But we do know that today we can stop and see the good around us. We can rejoice in our colleagues and their commitment with us to serving this community. We can give thanks for the patients and their families and the strength and courage they bring. There will be more than enough to worry about tomorrow, we know that for sure. But none of us have to face tomorrow alone. We can always call a meeting!

Amen.

9

Did You Hear the One About...?

Pleasant words are like a honeycomb, sweetness to the soul and health to the body.
Proverbs 16:24

When my husband and I were first married, twenty-seven short years ago, we were traditional starving students. We lived in St. Paul, Minnesota, where Steve was going to school. Our one night out was Saturday night. We would go around the corner to a tiny restaurant, slide into our regular booth, and order cheese pizza and one glass each of the house burgundy. After dinner we would drive downtown, park our rusty but trusty Toyota, and pay our fifty-cent admissions to the World Theater. Each week there would be a bake sale in the lobby, and we would buy a brownie to share. Then we would enter the darkened comfort of that cozy theater, sit down near the front, and watch a radio show being taped. It was tasty and expeditious.

Little did we know then that our favorite show and its wonderful host would become famous. We still listen to "Prairie Home Companion" on Minnesota Public Radio. Once a year or so, the host Garrison Keillor talks about jokes, complaining that because times are easier, people don't tell jokes like they did when he was growing up. He composes a ballad about the dearth of humor and then serves up a Saturday evening stew of stories and jokes. One year he included this medical one: "A man goes to the doctor with a frog on his head, and the doctor says, 'Where did you get that?' And the frog says, 'It started out as a little bump on my butt.'"

Well, I think Mr. Keillor is right about one thing and wrong about something else. He's right that people don't tell jokes like they used to. But he's wrong about things not being hard. Things are different, but they are often still very hard — especially in health care. I think this accounts for the trail of comics and clippings that end up taped to the doors or tacked to the bulletin boards of the offices of many healing people.

It is very easy to have a positive attitude in theory. I maintained a great outlook about a major renovation in the hospital in which I worked until I came back to my office and found a hole through the wall, caused by construction taking place next door. I tried to stay upbeat about it, but underneath I was exasperated. Lots of people try to project caring attitudes about others while working under difficult circumstances. Yet, together, with faith and a sense of humor, we are all making it through. It's a whole lot easier if we stick together.

Garrison Keillor's wisdom about the importance of humor is not anything new. The writer of the Old Testament book of Proverbs mentions this, too:

> *Anxiety weighs down the human heart,*
> *but a good word cheers it up.*
> **Proverbs 12:25**

> *A merry heart is a good medicine,*
> *but a downcast spirit dries up the bones.*
> **Proverbs 17:22**

So, I say to you — take care of one another. Tell each other jokes. Listen to one another's concerns. We are all in this together — and together, we will make it through the day. And we will be able to face tomorrow, come what may.

I leave you to consider one final medical case.

A lawyer is cross-examining a doctor about whether he had checked the pulse of the deceased before he signed the death certificate. "No," the doctor said, "I did not check his pulse." "And did you listen for a heartbeat?" said the lawyer. "No, I did not," said the doctor. "So," said the lawyer, "when you signed the death certificate, you had not taken steps to make sure he was dead." The doctor said, "Well, let me put it this way. The man's brain was in a jar on my desk, but for all I know he could still be out there practicing law somewhere."

Hang in there, and blessings!

Amen.

10

Showing Hospitality

Do not neglect to show hospitality to strangers, for by doing that some have entertained angels without knowing it.
Hebrews 13:2

When I arrived in the United States over thirty years ago to attend college, I was astonished by the reception I received. Everywhere on campus people said a word of greeting. I had grown up in a small town in Alberta, Canada, where almost everyone was related, and newcomers to the region (those who had been there less than fifty years) found that it took awhile to fit in. The hospitality I received from Americans was a completely new experience, one I have since had regularly over the many years I have lived here.

Healers are all about *hospitality* (from the same Latin root as "hospital" and "hospice"). Sometimes it is very difficult to show hospitality. There are so many competing demands. We often fall short of the mark — we forget someone, we can't be there for someone who needs us because another needs us more, we go on vacation and a patient or parishioner for whom we have cared has died. We work with real flesh and blood colleagues who often try our patience, just as we try theirs.

Father Daniel Homan, a member of the Order of St. Benedict, and Lonni Collins Pratt have authored *Radical Hospitality,* based on Benedictine spirituality and practice growing out of *The Rule of St. Benedict.* In this rich book, Fr. Homan and Ms. Pratt connect the messiness of modern life with the struggles of living in community — any community — family, work, faith community. They tell stories of wounds in relationships and stories of healing and acceptance of brokenness. One story they were given permission to share is from an episode in a friend's illness:

> When I was very ill, it was necessary to receive frequent intravenous treatments, injections, blood tests, and many intrusive medical treatments. At first I had the courage for it, but day after day I lost courage, until the day a small Korean woman, the head nurse, walked into my hospital room after several failed attempts to find a vein. I glared at her, pushed her hand away, and said, "I can't take this anymore."
>
> She nodded and held my hand, and we sat in the quiet for a minute or so. Then, she said, "I just finished injecting medication into a permanent port in the belly of a twelve-year-old boy who will probably die before the year is over. I could not take what I do if it weren't for the fact that sometimes what I do saves a life." I extended my arm and gave her my vein.[1]

Hospitality comes from a deep connection to God — from looking within and then reaching out even in the midst of chaos or conflict. This healer was able to overcome what was probably her initial reaction — that is, to shout, "You jerk! I just got through taking care of a twelve-year-old who probably will never live to see his teenage years, and you think you have problems?" Instead, she offered hospitality — starting with herself. She gave herself permission to examine her feelings as she held this patient's hand, and she took some quiet time to reflect. Only then was she was able to offer hospitality to her patient, who responded to her compassion. The sad but honest truth is, sometimes people won't respond to our best efforts. This is not a perfect world.

Indeed, our world faces so many challenges — war, economic woes, SARS, and all the "normal" diseases. Where do we find our peace? Our help comes from God, whose Spirit is ever present. We have a rich tradition of hospitality in our sacred texts and our religious pasts, if only we would take the time to read, to reflect, to ponder.

May we show hospitality in all that we do as healers. When we fall short of the mark (as we will), may we experience forgiving grace from God and from those we have failed in order to begin anew.

Amen!

11

The Woman with the CVA

Religion that is pure and undefiled before God is this: to visit orphans and widows in their affliction.
James 1:27a

Toward the end, she looked like every other person who had suffered a series of CVAs — cerebral vascular accidents, or "strokes." She sat in a chair, staring into space, turning her head from time to time in response to noise or speech, but seldom at the appropriate time so that one never knew whether she had comprehended. She looked tired, and anxious, and old.

Her hair was a shock of unruly white cotton — fine as spun silk. It was clean and combed and yet it was not the way she would have worn it, had she been able to do it herself. She wore a pretty blue and white floral housedress, ringed by a black lap belt, which kept her from sliding out of her chair.

She looked like the others around her. You wouldn't have picked her out for any particular reason. There wasn't much to know about her, based on her appearance. And yet....

She had been born in 1907 in a little village called Josefberg in what was then part of Austria, later Poland, now Ukraine. During WWII, soldiers threw a hand grenade into her family's house. The family remained safe, but the grenade blew up their sewing machine, a precious possession since her mother was a seamstress. They hid a Russian soldier behind a cupboard in their home to keep him from being killed by the Germans. She and her sisters had to drop out of school to work as domestic servants to help feed the family. She had less than a sixth-grade education.

She left Europe at twenty and sailed to the New World, with a promise from people in Canada that she could pay off the cost of the ticket by working for them. She did the work and paid off her passage. She married a young man in the community and they had a child. They farmed. They ran a blacksmith shop. They went to church. Her husband died. The child married and had three children of his own, whom she dearly loved. She grew older.

She had loved to put on an old pair of overalls, wrap a scarf around her hair, and go pick blueberries. She loved to work in the garden. She brought the dog and cats into her house in the winter when everyone else left their farm animals outside. She kept her home spotless, and she welcomed every visitor. She made cabbage rolls and potato-cheese dumplings and chocolate chip cookies by the ice-cream bucketful. Her house always smelled like a cross between sauerkraut and the dandelion wine she would make. She loved to sing in the church choir, and she genuinely enjoyed bingo. She could barely read, but "Under the B:14!" meant community to her on Friday nights. She could butcher a chicken or a pig or a cow with the best of them. She learned to crochet at a late age and gave everybody she knew afghans the colors of the rainbow. She knew about hope.

She's gone now. She was my grandma. I miss her.

I am grateful to those healing people who cared for my grandmother when she was sick. Some of them came to her funeral. They didn't know about the blueberries, or the church choir, or the sewing machine. They knew her only as Mrs. Krebs, an old woman who had suffered a series of CVAs. Yet they were so kind.

I am grateful to each person who plays a part in the care of other people's grandmas and grandpas. Mothers and fathers. Husbands and wives. Brothers and sisters and aunts and uncles and cousins and friends and lovers and children and neighbors. We touch so many lives when we care for the life of one. To feed someone, bathe them, clean their room, operate on them, pray for them — no matter what is done, that is a gift to that person and to all those who love her...or him.

Blessings to all who are healing people. May all that we do be done in a spirit of wisdom and compassion. May we offer the kindness of spirit we hope to receive when we ourselves are in need of care.

Amen and amen.

12

For Everything There is a Season?

For everything there is a season and a time for every matter under heaven.
Ecclesiastes 3:1

As I write this, the mercury in the thermometer is far below freezing. Some of the staff with whom I work had trouble starting their cars this morning. Our kitchen pipes have frozen under the dishwasher. The winter solstice is long past, yet due to the cold earth below, the air above has not yet embraced the warmth of the lengthening days. However, I know there is hope. As the writer of Ecclesiastes states, "For everything there is a season and a time for every matter under the heaven" (Ecclesiastes 3:1).

It is of course true that there is a time to be born, and a time to die, a time to be silent, and a time to speak. But, as healers, we often live in the gray areas between the clear-cut seasons.

Of course, there should be no season for rape and sexual harassment. There should be no season for sexual, physical, or emotional abuse of children, partners, or elders. There should be no season for the homeless to freeze, or the mentally ill to live in lonely isolation. There should be no season for living in such consumptive and unhealthy ways that millions of people in the Two-Thirds World do not have enough for basic needs.

We also struggle with more complex questions in our communal lives. Should there be a season for war? Certainly there should be no season for land mines or biological warfare. We seem to be living in a season of terrorism. Is there a role for healers to play in addressing international "dis-ease"?

We struggle with painful questions in our professional lives, and often come down on different sides of the issues. Even deciding on a course of treatment, or when to end treatment, can sometimes be debated. Sometimes we are faced with the question of how to respond when a colleague's choices may be putting others's well-being at risk. Ethical questions abound in the fields in which we work. We also struggle with painful questions in our personal lives, as diverse as we ourselves. What is the season? Is it a time to speak, or a time to keep silent?

As healers, first and foremost, we need to realize that we are not alone. We are working for and with the God of love, who calls us into relationship with one another. We are also working with other healers, each of whom is called to bring hope and healing to a wounded world. Our work stands on the shoulders and insights of others who have gone before. We are not alone.

Paradoxically, as healers, we also need to realize that we are alone. We, individually, are responsible for each professional judgment that we make. As James R. Lowell wrote in 1845 during the build-up to the Mexican-American War:

> *Once to every man and nation, comes the moment to decide,*
> *in the strife of truth with falsehood, for the good or evil side;*
> *some great cause, some great decision, offering each the bloom*
> *or blight,*
> *and the choice goes by forever, 'twixt that darkness and*
> *that light.*[1]

There are times when we must make hard choices. Will we live in a season of courage? Will we live in a season of risk? Will we live in a season of hope? Will we recognize the season to die?

When we have struggled with the questions and found answers for the seasons that bring healing and hope, we can give thanks and move on. We must recognize, however, that the seasons continue to change, and we must continue to seek new answers.

Medicine is always seeking new answers, new truths. Theology has not always been so willing to explore the ever-changing cosmos. This may be one of the greatest reasons for the huge split that has arisen in the last century between medicine and theology. Lowell wrote:

> *New occasions teach new duties, time makes*
> *ancient good uncouth,*
> *They must upward still and onward, who would*
> *keep abreast of truth.*[2]

Healers need each other, to learn from the wisdom of those who have gone before and to hear the prophetic words of those who would call us onward. Healers also need to spend some time alone, for personal reflection and wrestling with the gray days found in every season. We all need to keep learning, to keep asking questions. No one has all the answers — we all need to be open to change and the possibility that we might be wrong. For we will be wrong, at times.

The world needs all its healers. We need to find seasons of healing for ourselves. The world needs all our energy, all our work. We do not know when a word as an advocate or prophet will change a heart or a mind. We do not know when a particular intervention will make all the difference in a person's life or all the difference in the world. We should not grow weary in well-doing. As you minister to and with those in your communities, know that new seasons are always coming. Each new season brings days of sorrow and days of joy, and many, many days that are somewhere in between.

The writer of Ecclesiastes also says, "I know that there is nothing better for people than to be happy and do good while they live" (Ecclesiastes 3:12). Maybe that is why God is calling so many as healers. Be happy. Do good. For doing good is always in season, perhaps carrying happiness along the way.

Blessings, and amen.

13

Stewards of God's Mysteries

This is how one should regard us, as servants of Christ and stewards of the mysteries of God.
1 Corinthians 4:1

At the International Parish Nurse Resource Center, we get a number of calls from the press. They ask, "How many parish nurses are there? What does a parish nurse do?"

Generally, I answer their questions, and then I start telling them the stories. I tell them about Claudia Golliday, who not only worked with traumatized Afghani women refugees, but who left her comfortable suburban home and moved into the inner-city neighborhood to be near them. I tell them about Joyce Lony, a parish nurse who also leads an Interfaith Volunteer Caregivers organization, providing support to the most vulnerable and alone. I tell them about Eileen McCartland, who works with a great number of mentally ill neighbors near the inner-city cathedral where she is a parish nurse. I tell them about Linda Stoeklin, who has a prayer shawl ministry, providing sheltering comfort to the grieving and afflicted. I tell them about Beth Durban, whose health fairs regularly draw large crowds and include most of the health providers in the region. I tell them about Mary Ann Brischetto, who has helped over 200 fragile inner-city families and who has state legislators calling her — on her cell phone. I tell them about Becky Valicoff, who waited outside a church neighbor's house, in the middle of the night, during an arrest for domestic violence. When the police left, she helped the woman then and in the months that followed. I tell them about Nadine Davis, who started a food pantry and clothing exchange in one of the poorest neighborhoods in town. And that's just some of what is happening in St. Louis. I tell them about Chicago, and Virginia, and Iowa, and Wisconsin, and Seattle, and Arizona, and Canada, and Australia, and New Zealand, and Korea, and Swaziland. And I tell them about Sister Bena.

Sister Bena was a Deaconess Sister who lived in St. Louis during World War I. She worked at Caroline Mission, serving a community about two or three miles southwest of downtown St. Louis. Sister Bena visited the sick and homebound, and arranged access to a physician or the hospital for those whose conditions required it. She helped feed "hobos," as the homeless were called then. She sought jobs for the unemployed, in a time before welfare, Social Security, or pensions. She taught sewing classes, led a mothers' group, distributed secondhand clothes, and gave talks to churches and women's fellowship groups to raise funds for the mission.

Here are a few entries from the journal of Sister Bena's assistant for a few days in 1914:

> **April 29:** Home calls on Mr. and Mrs. Nelson Leriche. Mrs. L. very weak. Teachers Meeting in evening. Stayed with Mrs. L during the night, and cared for conditions at the home — Mrs. L. very much neglected — great disorder — dirt and bugs.
>
> **May 2:** Mrs. Leriche passed away early Saturday morning. Sister Bena was called to the Leriche home and was asked to make the shroud, Mr. L. bringing the goods for same to sewing-school. The shroud was made Saturday night.
>
> **May 3:** Sunday School. Sister Bena taking shroud to Leriche.
>
> **May 4:** Funeral of Mrs. Leriche. Beautiful flowers, many friends! After the funeral, made home visits on Bonre, Most, and Potter.
>
> **May 5:** Cleaning the hall. Home visits to Vageder, Wall, Gerding, Moore (a member of Centenary Church), Ronik, Crabtree.[1]

Sister Bena's world was very different from today and yet so very similar. There are still individuals and families falling through the cracks who need help. Parish nurse Josephine Fields recently made a home visit to the family of a little girl with whom she worked. The child, who was in an after-school class, couldn't read at all, even though she was eight. What Josephine found when she got there was a young, overwhelmed, single mom with five kids. The oldest, aged nine, was doing well at home and in school. The younger school-aged children, however, were not yet enrolled in school because their mother did not have their immunizations up-to-date and copies of their birth certificates. Josephine loaded the family in her car and helped the mother get the kids immunized. She helped them get their birth certificates and helped them sign up for school That little girl is now reading. Is that a health issue? In fact, it is! Low educational status generally is a predictor of poor future health. Where does Josephine minister? In exactly the same neighborhood where Sister Bena worked nearly 100 years ago.

The Greek word that Paul used for "steward" is "oikonomos." (It sounds like the word "economics" and shares the same root.) It was the word used for a manager or steward of a household in ancient times. We are called to be stewards of God's household.

You — nurses, doctors, and clergy working in hospitals or churches — are those stewards. And you, like all the saints, are equipped with what you need to do your work.

First, a steward needs compassion. It is hard to do this work unless you genuinely care about people. Luckily, compassion is a trait shared by almost all those who are attracted to the healing professions. It is challenged, however, by the conditions of health-care delivery today. Many healers suffer terribly from compassion fatigue. It is not because they never had compassion; it is because their compassion has been entirely used up.

Second, a steward needs courage. It takes guts to do this work. You are working with the sick and the suffering, and they often complain and whine and, many times, dang it, they are contagious.

Third, a steward needs creativity. A good steward is constantly thinking of ways to improve the running of the household. A good steward is thinking

Stewards of God's Mysteries

of ways to encourage the rest of the household to work together.

Finally, the stewards of God's mysteries need to pray. Healers need to be filled with living water as they come to the wellsprings of God's love and are renewed and strengthened, finding the comfort of knowing that they are not alone.

Healers are called as stewards of the mysteries of God. They work with the tools of compassion, courage, creativity, and prayer. They work with the mysteries of Body. They walk with the mysteries of Soul. They live within the temporal and the eternal, the earthly and the transcendent.

Remember your roots. Remember your stories. Remember your sacred commission. You are called, you are named, and you are needed as stewards of the mysteries of God.

Amen and amen.

14

Life is What Happens...

A time to be born, and a time to die.
Ecclesiastes 3:2a

Not long ago, my father-in-law died. He was a Presbyterian minister who inspired me to enter the ministry, and had spent a lot of time with us and our children, especially during the all-too-few years since his retirement. His death was expected, yet it was still a blow. Our trips to visit him as he was dying and again for the funeral shifted us all behind in work and school.

Why I am telling you this? Because life happens smack-dab in the middle of other life, and death is a part of that life. Because what each of us has on our schedule for one day may not be what we accomplish that day. Because we, as family members, doctors, nurses, clergy, or other health professionals, are responsible for so much, to so many, in so many different settings.

Healers walk with pregnant mothers, dying grandfathers, runaway teenagers, and stubborn middle-aged men (who don't want to go to the doctor unless they have no choice). They hear stories of journeys through great pain and empathize as patients or parishioners share fears. They listen, and they listen, and they listen. Only then do they speak, only then do they act. But always, if you want to be an effective healer, you must also do something else that you most likely were taught *not* to do: You must feel.

Henry James, the nineteenth-century American author who wrote such classics as *Portrait of a Lady, Daisy Miller,* and *The Bostonians,* wrote in a letter to Clare Sheridan, a friend whose newlywed husband was sent off to war in 1915, "Feel, feel, I say — feel for all you're worth, and even if it half kills you, for that is the only way to live, especially to live at this terrible pressure, and the only way to honor and celebrate these admirable beings who are our pride and our inspiration."[1]

A healer who is totally caught up in every emotional battle of a patient or parishioner will soon be of no value to anyone. But a healer who is unable to feel the pain of any wounds will also be of no value to anyone. We need to embrace the unexpected and allow in both pain and joy. For in doing so, we will fully experience the presence of those with whom we live and work, and also the presence of God. And that is the only way to live, especially at this terrible pressure.

Amen.

15

The Healing Power of the Ordinary

Blessed are those who hunger and thirst for righteousness, for they shall be satisfied.
Matthew 5:6

First, you take a cup of whipping cream and a half-pound of white chocolate. Bring the cream to a boil and melt the chocolate into the cream. Set this sauce aside. Then take three cups of whipping cream, a cup of whole milk, and a half-cup of sugar. Stir them together in a saucepan and heat until the sugar dissolves. Add the other half-pound of chocolate and whisk until melted. Slowly add, already beaten, eight egg yolks and two whole eggs. Add a cut-up loaf of French bread and stir. Put this into a baking dish, cover, and bake for an hour. Put re-warmed sauce and berries over it. Now you have white chocolate bread pudding. It has only 4,700 calories per serving.

Now I know that this recipe has more cholesterol than biscuits and gravy, a double cheeseburger, and toasted ravioli all rolled together. So why did I give it to you? It's not a special day like Easter, or Thanksgiving, or Christmas. Ah, but it is a special day! It is a day for which you may have plans — perhaps to work, perhaps to be with friends, perhaps to relax at home. It *is* a very special day — an ordinary day! There is great healing power in the ordinary.

Now of course, when a person needs a heart transplant, he/she doesn't want the ordinary. He/she wants the most extraordinary healers in charge. Most of what people generally need in order to be whole, however, is ordinary — clean water, nutritious food, vigorous exercise, restful sleep, celebration with friends, and time for spiritual pursuits. It is in the ordinary that we can be sustained and renewed. It is in the ordinary that we can touch the transcendent.

We find healing and purpose in the ordinary, I believe, when we see the ordinary as the place where the sacred dwells with us. John Ellerton, in 1890, wrote a hymn for a midday service in an urban church, in which he says of God,

> *The chapel's not the only place your presence may be found;*
> *On daily work you shed your grace, and blessings all abound.*
> *Yours are the workplace, home, and mart, the wealth*
> *   of sea and land;*
> *The worlds of science and of art are fashioned by your hand.*[1]

If we take just a moment to experience a sense of the sacred in what we do, we can experience the healing power of the ordinary. Healers are part of a tradition of work and renewal in ordinary time. We follow those who lived out their prayers in their ordinary lives. John Ellerton writes, in the last verse of his hymn,

> *Work shall be prayer, if all be wrought as you would*
> *   have it done;*
> *And prayer, by you inspired and taught, shall then*
> *   with work be one.*[2]

You don't have to have white chocolate bread pudding for dinner to celebrate this day. But you *can*. See the sacred in each ordinary moment, and greet the sacred in each person whose life you touch.

Amen.

16

Time and Chance Happen to Us All

Again I see that under the sun the race is not to the swift, nor the battle to the strong, nor bread to the wise, nor riches to the intelligent, nor favor to the men of skill, but time and chance happen to them all.
Ecclesiastes 9:11-12

Late last summer, there was a wonderful commercial on television. It showed a father pushing a shopping cart through an office supply store, followed by several children. He was smiling broadly and skipping as he tossed school supplies into his cart. In the background a voice was singing, "It's the Most Wonderful Time of the Year!" Ah, the beginning of the school year!

Having been associated with the beginnings of school years for over forty years now, first as a student, later as the wife of a seminary professor, now as the mother of two school-aged children, I do find September the most wonderful time of the year. It is refreshing to revel in the season of school supplies, of moving vans bringing new seminary students from near and far. It is the time of college students carting loads of yet-unopened textbooks and wearing their newest finery. Ah, beginnings! Fresh starts, unbounded hope, uncharted waters, the future stretching out for miles ahead. A most wonderful time of life. What a *precious* time of life — and how quickly it flies by!

They say that time slows as you approach the speed of light. My own theory is that at more mundane speeds, time accelerates. From the vantage point of my forty-some years, it seems that childhood lasts about half an hour, then there is about an hour until middle age. After that there is about an hour until retirement, and then forty-five minutes to an hour left if we are lucky. The way I see it, college students have about two hours until they retire.

"Time and chance happen to them all." The person who wrote the words of this text from Ecclesiastes has long since come and gone. In this writing we can hear the words of one who was both wise and realistic. This woman or man had seen it all and knew that her or his life, like grass, would soon be gone. This writer saw the vanity and futility of much of life and thought the best way to spin through this world was by enjoying it responsibly. Like many Jewish theologians of that day, the writer did not believe in life after death. This is it, so you better make the most of life's brief span. Time and chance happen to us all.

When I woke up one recent morning, I looked outside to see our recycling bin and milk jugs gone, and just a pile of tin cans lying there. When we went out to investigate, we found that someone had burned the bin. Now, we live near a seminary in a neighborhood where one would not expect vandalism. It looked like gasoline had been poured into the bin, however, to consume it so completely. All that remained were a few twisted scraps of matted, green plastic. The grass was charred, but thanks to recent rain, the flames hadn't spread further.

It was futile to ask who might have started this fire. I couldn't think of anyone who had something against us, so it must have been one of those random acts of senseless vandalism teenagers are prone to on a frisky spring night before graduation.

We have all experienced such random events, which, by mere chance, affect us. Some are very small, like losing a possession that holds some meaning or usefulness for us. Some are huge — like the terrible tsunami that occurred near the end of 2004, killing so many in Southeast Asia and Indonesia. We know that no one is singled out by the universe for such pain. Time and chance happen to us all.

The thought that time is passing quickly and that chance plays a role in our lives can be either comforting or terribly worrying. Holding the knowledge close that time passes quickly enriches the time we have together. Can anyone look at a baby and not think how quickly that time passes? Can anyone look at an elderly parent and not wonder about the years left together? And what if something should happen? Each moment is so precious.

The writer of Ecclesiastes is not saying that we shouldn't bother to run the race of this earthly life because something bad might happen. We have to try and give the race our best shot. What he or she is saying, however, is don't beat yourself up if you are not famous, or rich, or powerful, and don't give up your spirit if you are not free from hardship or tragedy because you can still have a rich and full life. Time and chance happen to us all.

Time and chance happened to the family of Bertha and Harry Holt. During the depression they lost their home in South Dakota and moved to Oregon to start over again. They worked hard, and by the 1950s they were the parents of six children and owned a prosperous lumber, farming, and fishing business. One day, while hiking into a stand of timber, Harry suffered a massive heart attack. As he was convalescing, the Holts happened to see a TV documentary about orphans created by the Korean War. Right then and there, the Holts decided to adopt as many Korean orphans as they could. The only problem was, intercountry adoption was then not allowed. It would take an act of Congress to change that. "We'll do it," said Bertha, and in a few months, the law was changed. In 1955 Harry escorted home eight children from Korea. In 1956, the next year, the family started the Holt Adoption Agency, which has helped to find homes for thousands of orphans from countries around the globe. Harry died in 1964, only nine years after bringing home the children from Korea. But Bertha, known as "Grandma Holt" by then, carried on. She was still running a mile a day when she died of a stroke in 1994, thirty years later.

Life is a precious adventure, meant to be savored and to be experienced to the fullest, with compassion and empathy for others. Time and chance happen to us all. Who knows what life holds in store for any of us on any given day? But we need not fear meaninglessness, even if tragedy should strike. For whatever happens to us in life, we always have the choice to live openly to others, focusing on relationships and caring. We can embrace those causes that feed our soul. We can give ourselves to communities in which we are cared for and where we can find ways to care for others.

Amen and amen.

17

Jesus, the Great Healer

They brought him all the sick, those afflicted with various diseases and pain, demoniacs, epileptics, and paralytics, and he healed them.
Matthew 4:24b

A few years ago, right before Christmas, my husband had to go to a hospital emergency department. Steve had been playing basketball, and a sharp undercut to his jaw took him by surprise. The impact brought his teeth sharply together, unfortunately, catching his tongue mid-bite. He drove himself to the hospital for stitches.

In the Emergency Department, time always seems long for patients. While he was there, he heard the doctor give a rundown of the patients who were there. "Let's see, 'The Heart' is in that room, 'The Ankle' is in there, and 'The Tongue" is down the hall." (Now with HIPAA, these patients would be called "The Chest," "The Leg," and "The Head" to avoid revealing sensitive health information.)

At the time, Steve thought, "A four-year bachelor's degree, two master's degrees, and an expensive Ph.D., for which I am still paying, and I'm reduced to 'The Tongue.'"

Well, at least The Tongue had health insurance. He showed his card, which displayed the amount of his co-pay. Pity the Tongues who have no insurance. They are stabilized and sent on their way, or treated and charged a rate far higher than that charged the Insured Tongue.

And his skin was the right color. There is much data to show that Tongues who come in surrounded by anything but off-white skin have a harder time being treating in Emergency or any other department. Same goes for their treatment in the church.

And The Tongue was of the right gender. Too often the health concerns of women are treated less seriously, particularly if they present their health concern as related to The Heart.

Four hours later, The Tongue was discharged. It was Christmastime, and the only thing that the guy could eat was Ensure®. And The Tongue didn't talk too well, either, so even people who had known him (and taught with him on the same seminary faculty) started talking to him like he was profoundly retarded. His intellectual abilities weren't impacted one bit that day, but for weeks he was treated very differently by strangers and friends.

We have heard Jesus called the Great Physician, but he was also the Great Nurse and the Great Rabbi. Jesus listened. He wasn't on an HMO-prescribed limit of eight- to twelve-minutes-per-patient appointment, seeing only those who were covered by the plan his office accepted. He wasn't trying to finish all his paperwork before the shift change. Jesus listened to the stories of people who were suffering, and he did all that he could to help them. He gave from the heart. He touched people's lives when they were scared and vulnerable — women, men, Jews, Gentiles — all who came to him.

Jesus taught. He told stories and parables to give people the vision they needed to change their lives — to change their behaviors, their habits, their beliefs — to bring them healing and wholeness. Healers teach all the time — helping people to change their health practices. Jesus was a counselor, an advocate for the weak, a comforter, and a challenger.

It takes courage to be a healer today. It is challenging to welcome the sick. Modern diseases like AIDS or SARS are frightening, and they represent risk to the healer. Serving as a healer will always be a challenging form of caring for others. Yet you have risen to that challenge, and you have agreed that you will care for people in body, mind, and spirit — as whole people. You teach them, touch them, and go to where they are. You set forth each day to change the world, by healing it one person at a time.

Live your own stories to the fullest. Listen to the stories of those for whom you care. Go forth, dear friends, with God's blessing, and know that you are called to a ministry of love and care, just as God loves and cares for you.

Amen.

18

The Empire of Healing

And Jesus went about all the cities and villages, teaching in their synagogues and preaching the gospel of the kingdom, and healing every disease and every infirmity.
Matthew 9:35

I love Lent! I love the fact that it is one of the few church observances that the greeting card industry has not yet exploited. You will not find any lenten merchandise in the stores. I think there *would* be cards, but nobody in the industry is entirely certain what ideas you can sell for Lent. "Happy Repentance!" "Joyous Imposition of Ashes!" I just don't know.

So, what is Lent to healers? It consists of the forty days before Easter, excluding Sundays, which are always feast days. It commemorates the last days of Jesus' life and culminates in Good Friday, the day of his death. Perhaps the meaning of Lent can be found there.

We don't really know exactly what happened in the forty days before Jesus was crucified, despite the books and movies that attempt to tell us. We know about some of the events surrounding his crucifixion. We know that he celebrated Passover with his friends. Legend tells us that a woman poured expensive oil over him, to comfort and sustain him, and to prepare him for martyrdom. We know that he prayed alone a great deal, and that he spoke to many crowds. We know that he was aware of a growing resentment by the authorities of his ministry of healing and inclusion.

Maybe a key to Lent is to look at why Jesus was killed. Jesus lived in a Jewish land, occupied by the Roman Empire. The Jews were allowed their customs and their worship as long as they didn't challenge the authority of

Caesar. And there was Jesus, preaching about another empire. He was saying that the Empire of God was here! He was saying, "Give Caesar what is Caesar's and give God what is God's" (Mark 12:17). The Jewish people knew their scriptures. "The earth is the Lord's, and the fullness thereof" (Psalm 24:1). In that worldview, there was nothing that belonged to Caesar. No allegiance is owed a sovereign who rules by terror and extortion.

In proclaiming a new empire, Jesus turned to those for whom the Roman Empire had little use. He said, "Blessed are you poor, for yours is the empire of God" (Luke 6:20b). He fed the hungry and embraced the outcasts. He talked with the mentally ill and reminded them that they were whole in the eyes of God. He healed lepers and called them back into God's community when he knew that this would make him unclean. He touched and healed bleeding women when he knew that it would defile him. He proclaimed an empire for all those dispossessed and discouraged by the imperial ordering of his world, and so he became an imperial enemy. What got him killed was his rock-solid belief that the earth is the Lord's, not the emperor's. We belong to God. Our lives do not belong to the Roman Empire, the British Empire, or the multinational corporate empires. The work of healing does not belong to the hospitals, the HMOs, or the health insurance empires. It belongs to us — we who believe in the goodness and everlasting love of God, and who believe in the right of all people to partake in that healing goodness. Such thinking probably won't get you killed today, but it might still make you an enemy of the empire.

God is calling many of those who would heal and be healed to embrace both reflection and action during the season of Lent. We are called to reflect on the love of God and to see how that love is to be borne out through our lives and our ministries. We are called to advocate for the sick, the lonely, and the outcast. We are called to measure our lives against the standard of love and acceptance that Jesus set. We are called to prayer, and to repentance, with only one goal: to learn that God loves us and calls us into community in the empire that has no end.

Amen.

19

The Church's Call to Health Ministry

When Jesus saw the crowds, he had compassion for them, because they were harassed and helpless, like sheep without a shepherd. Then he said to his disciples, "The harvest is plentiful, but the laborers are few; pray therefore the Lord of the harvest to send out laborers into his harvest."
Matthew 9:36-38

In a church I served, probably very much like the church you serve or attend, there were people who got sick. Sometimes they would need to go to the hospital. The hospital would take care of them for a few days, then send them back home. Often the hospital would call me and ask if we had anyone in the church who could help at home.

We also had homebound members with health concerns. Sometimes people needed to move into nursing homes, and it was hard for their families to find the right place. Some folks had illnesses that were misdiagnosed, and advocating for another opinion got them the help they needed. A church community often has many health-related concerns. So when I was offered the opportunity to serve on the board of a large health system in St. Louis, I jumped at the chance. I thought, "Oh boy, here's my chance to change how health care interacts with the church."

I learned more about how hospitals are run as well as some of the myriad regulations under which they operate. I learned more about the economic and social complexities of hospital administration. For example, I learned more about how health insurance works. I learned that some insurance companies pay the full charges on a hospital's bill. But those companies providing that kind of indemnity insurance are now few and far between. Most companies pay a negotiated rate that is lower than the total bill. Often it is a great deal lower, sometimes by more than half. There are many other strategies some health insurance companies use to maximize their profits, too numerous and ever-changing to list here.

Needless to say, I learned a lot during my years on the health-system board. There are few clear-cut lines between good guys and bad guys in health care. And the current health-care system we have is primarily an "illness care" system, if it can even be called a "system" at all.

There is an old eastern European parable that I heard some time ago. It goes something like this:

There was a man who had a dream. In that dream, he finds a priceless treasure buried under the bridge in Prague. So he travels to Prague, finds the bridge, and frantically begins to dig. As he is digging, a guard approaches, stops him, and asks him what he is doing. The man tells the guard of his curious dream. The guard laughs and tells him that he, too has had a dream of treasure the night before. He had dreamed that he would find a fool digging for treasure under the bridge, but in reality the treasure was under his own house. So the man returns home and digs beneath his own stones. There he finds the dreamed-of treasure.

Not too long ago, the Centers for Disease Control and Prevention released some interesting figures. They had done research to learn what impact our health system has upon a person's health status. What they learned was rather startling. They found that 50 percent of the factors impacting health are related to one's lifestyle, 20 percent are related to one's immediate environment, and 20 percent are related to genetics. That adds up to 90 percent. Only 10 percent of the factors impacting health are related to the health-care delivery system. It is for this 10 percent that our nation spends 15 percent of its gross national product.

Research done by Drs. Ron and Janice Glaser of Ohio State University in Columbus, Ohio, found that the factor most likely to negatively affect the immune system was loneliness.[1] Other studies have shown that people who participate in faith communities are less likely to abuse alcohol or drugs. Still other studies show that an active prayer life contributes to a healthier life.

The "Nun Study" conducted by the National Institute on Aging showed higher mental functioning among religious elderly women than among the general elderly population.

Here's the irony. I left the church to go into hospital work to try and fix the health system in my community, but in reality one could make a much larger impact on health and wellness through a congregation. Hospitals can't fix loneliness. Churches can. Hospitals usually can't keep in close contact with people long enough to change their personal health habits. Churches can. Hospitals can't mentally, socially, emotionally, and spiritually engage people on a regular basis for years. Churches can.

There is treasure right under our noses. Churches can bring lonely people back into the community and heal their loneliness. Churches can help educate people about environmental health concerns. Churches in a community can band together and make it tough for kids to have access to cigarettes. They can impact housing codes and make certain that people live in safe housing. I know churches in rural communities often advocate for safe water, and many parishioners there grow healthy food for themselves and others.

Parishioners working together can make a community a healthier place to live. We certainly need hospitals for treatment of serious illnesses or injuries. Few would choose to live in a community without a good hospital. That is the reason that churches started most of the hospitals in this country. Faith communities started hospitals all around the world.

Today, the church is reclaiming an important role in promoting health and wholeness. It has always believed that it had a part to play in spiritual health, but it also has a profound ability to influence physical and mental health. Those in the church are called to heal the sick, bind up the broken-hearted, and proclaim the healing and life-transforming love of God.

Amen.

20

Gender as a Health Issue

So God created man in his own image, in the image of God he created him; male and female he created them.
Genesis 1:27

The scene is a courtroom filled with lawyers and witnesses. The accused stands before the judge to hear the verdict as it is announced. The judge speaks. "You are charged with a serious offense. Your appearance has brought pain to your family. Because of you, your family fears poverty. Because of you, your parents fear abandonment in old age. Because of you, your parents fear the possibility of dishonor. Because of you, your family is forced to make hard choices.

"You have been found guilty," the judge continues. "The sentence is death. There are no options for appeal."

"But I have done nothing wrong!" the accused cries out. "I have done nothing at all! Of what crime am I guilty?"

The judge sighs. This was an old story. A very old story, one that the judge had heard many, many times, in many, many places. And very often the same verdict is handed down: the death sentence. The judge speaks quietly.

"You are guilty," the judge says, "of coming into this world as a girl child."

When I recently participated in a symposium on the girl child in India, I was on sabbatical there and knew little about what I assumed was an obscure topic. What I learned was astonishing.

I read newspaper accounts describing the marriages of very young girl children to teenagers or older men. I read stories of bride-burnings, setting women on fire, for want of "adequate" dowries. I read about a young woman who seemed to have it all, the former Miss India, Nafisa Joseph, who committed suicide because her marriage had been called off. I read about girls held captive by circuses, to be used as sex workers. I read about girls sold by their parents because of desperate financial straits. Usually they are sold into brothels in Mumbai (Bombay) or Kolcuta (Calcutta) or any number of other cities where they service men for 30 rupees (less than a dollar) a turn. They work to pay off debts that continually mount and will never be repaid.

But another alarming story in India and other impoverished countries is more subtle. It is the story of the declining ratio of girls to boys. At a rally in New Delhi on July 10, 2004, Narayan Banerjee, director of the Centre for Women's Development Studies in Delhi, addressed the crowd. She shared statistics that showed that only about 865 girls per 1,000 boys are born in Delhi because of the preferential sex selection of boys over girls through abortion. Those who are unable to afford amniocentesis and an abortion and still wish to select for boys must resort to female infanticide. Banerjee pleads, "It is important that awareness about female infanticide should be translated into action. We also need to seek help from the medical fraternity, the source from which female infanticide happens so that we can tackle the problem more effectively."[1]

So I turned to Indian literature to find signs of hope there. What I found were books like *Come Up and Be Dead* by prominent Bangalore writer Shashi Deshpande.

In this novel, her protagonist Kshama is bewildered at the birth of her brother and at her father's (Appa's) enormous pride in the event. Desphande writes, "Kshama had been sixteen when Pratap was born. It had seemed a disaster to her.... 'My son....' The way Appa had said those words somehow diminished her. It had struck terror in her. 'Don't I matter at all? Don't I count any more?'"[2]

In her award-winning novel *Mistaken Identity,* Nayantara Sahgal writes about a young man learning about the methods used for killing girl babies. "There are methods of strangling with the umbilical cord. Another popular method was a pill of *bhang.* Very safe and simple this was. The midwife put the pill on the infant's tongue and it slid down the throat like a sweetie, or she smeared the mother's nipple with it and the infant swallowed it with the first suck. However, if they buried the infant alive as some did, first they filled the hole up tenderly with milk.... It did start me wondering if the two girl children Mother had had before me had been stillborn after all, or lay buried in milky holes under ground I bicycled over every day."[3]

Deshpande, Sahgal, Banerjee — surely they exaggerate the situation. No, says the Rev. Solomon Benjamin, a senior executive with the YMCA in India. He says that often the mother of a girl child is forced to kill the girl by her mother-in-law, who does not want her son to have to bear the financial burden of a daughter. The twin evils of poverty and sexism combine to put the girl child at risk the moment her gender is discovered.

Of course, the concern for the welfare of the girl child is not limited to India. In China, the orphanages are filled with girls. It seems that when you have but one child to keep, many prefer that it be a boy. Girl children in China are killed through methods similar to those used in India and other poor countries. In a recent interview with Bill Moyer, Shirley Goek-Lin reports that "one of the favorite ways of killing these little baby girls is to turn their faces over in soot. Soot is readily available in peasant homes, and you don't have to reuse it. You can throw it out with the infant." Her "Pantoun for Chinese Women" sends chills down the spine. She writes, "At present, the phenomena of butchering, drowning and leaving to die female infants have been very serious" (*The People's Daily*, Peking, March 3, 1983).

> *They say a child with two mouths is no good.*
> *In the slippery wet, a hollow space,*
> *Smooth, gumming, echoing wide for food.*
> *No wonder my man is not here at his place.*
>
> *In this slippery wet, a hollow space,*
> *A slit narrowly sheathed within its hood.*
> *No wonder my man is not here at his place:*
> *He is digging for the dragon jar of soot.*

That slit narrowly sheathed within its hood!
His mother, squatting, coughs by the fire's blaze
While he digs for the dragon jar of soot.
We had saved for a hundred days.

His mother, squatting, coughs by the fire's blaze.
The child kicks against me mewing like a flute.
We had saved ashes for a hundred days.
Knowing, if the time came, that we would.

The child kicks against me crying like a flute
Through its two weak mouths. His mother prays
Knowing when the time comes that we would,
For broken clay is never set in glaze.

Through her two weak mouths his mother prays.
She will not pluck the rooster nor serve its blood,
For broken clay is never set in glaze:
Women are made of river sand and wood.

She will not pluck the rooster nor serve its blood.
My husband frowns, pretending in his haste
Women are made of river sand and wood.
Milk soaks the bedding. I cannot bear the waste.

My husband frowns, pretending in his haste.
Oh clean the girl, dress her in ashy soot!
Milk soaks our bedding, I cannot bear the waste.
They say a child with two mouths is no good.[4]

Poverty and sexism are deadly to women and girls in the Third World. But sexism affects women's health everywhere. Women bear the largest load for housework, care of children, and elderly parents in every land, even if they work full-time elsewhere, often at risk to their own well-being. A recent survey by the National Women's Health Resource Center found that nearly 95 percent of all adult women sleep less than eight hours per night. Women's health issues are not priorities for researchers. The world is not yet a place of equality for women, in any land.

Then one day I picked up the Bangalore daily newspaper, the *Deccan Herald,* and read about an abandoned girl baby in Lucknow, India. At least fifteen families offered to adopt her. According to the story, "Femida Bano, mother of five boys and one of the many who offered to adopt the girl explains, 'Daughters are precious and only the blessed have them.'"[5]

A few years ago, Geeta Rathore was elected to leadership in her village in Madhya Pradesh. Because of her leadership, every girl child in her village now goes to school, and every woman has become a member of a self-help group, with her own bank account and income. We know that education and improved financial situations are prime factors in the improvement of maternal and child health in every country. But before these things can happen for women and girls, people of wisdom must begin to challenge sexism wherever it exists — in Bangalore, Beijing, or Boston.

In the time of Christian origins the sages of Israel read Genesis 1:27 and realized that God knows no gender. When the first Christians were baptized they were made to know that in Christ there is "no male and female" (Galatians 3:28). Let us pray that in this world made by God, all girls and women, boys and men, will be allowed the good portion — life, and a chance to live it. For we are all — men and boys, women and girls — made in the "image of God." This is ancient wisdom, and it is wisdom indeed.

Amen.

21

Seeking the Sabbath

A time to keep, and a time to cast away.
Ecclesiastes 3:6b

If you would have looked in my office recently, you would have seen sorting, filing, and pitching. This is not because I enjoy sorting, filing, and pitching. It is because I was feeling paralyzed by my ever-growing list of "Things to Do." Nearly every healer with whom I speak mentions this trend — there is always more to be done. None of us can do it alone!

Thankfully, there are ways through the maze of hurry with which most of us are well familiar. One way is to stop and take time to be with family, friends, and God.

Our society has wandered far from the biblical concept of "Sabbath." Stores remain open on Sundays, sports teams practice and play, and there are always errands to run that never seem to get done during the week.

God reminds us, through taking time for prayer and meditation and for Sabbath worship, rest and renewal, that fully completing our work is an illusion. We are called to participate in God's work, but we will never be able to accomplish everything we would like. We are to rest secure in the thought that if we follow in God's ways, our work will be blessed, and it will be enough.

What price does our society pay for this task-focus marathon? We work more hours than any other nation on earth. We eat fast food, and we export it to other countries, even though it is filled with salt, fat, and simple carbohydrates. We are sleep-deprived, and our kids are suffering. *The New York Times* stated that the group of Americans with the largest increase in antidepressant use between 1998 and 2002 was preschool children — an increase of over

50 percent.[1] College students are experiencing stress at ever greater levels.[2] We are living in "Never" Land: Never take a break.

Wayne Muller, the founder of Bread for the Journey, a nonprofit that provides funds for social services in impoverished neighborhoods, has recently written *Sabbath: Finding Rest, Renewal, and Delight in our Busy Lives*. He writes, "Sabbath time is not spiritually superior to our work. The practice is rather to find that balance point at which, having rested, we do our work with greater ease and joy, and bring healing and delight to our endeavors. Even if we were to leave work behind and seek the comfort and security of a monastery, we would be handed a broom, and told to sweep the walks.... But there is a time to sweep, and a time to put down the broom and rest."[3] May you, too, embrace time to work, rest, and play.

Amen and amen.

22

I Like Your Shoes

If the whole body were an eye, where would be the hearing? If the whole body were an ear, where would be the sense of smell?"
I Corinthians 12:17

One interesting thing about working with health and ministry professionals is seeing the type of shoes they wear. I've seen all kinds. I've seen sneakers and heels. White support shoes and black oxfords. Comfy slip-ons and sturdy lace-ups. Steel-toed work boots and those little blue paper booties that go over shoes in surgery. Keds and Nikes and Reeboks and Easy Spirits. Lots of Easy Spirits in health care.

Patients don't often notice them. When you are behind a desk, they can't see your shoes. When patients are lying in bed, they certainly can't see your shoes. But they always see who fills them.

These shoes are filled by people who care about others. They are people who care about their work. The shoes in the worlds of healing are filled with people who work hard. Their shoes cover a lot of miles most days. If you added together all the miles covered by all the employees in a single hospital for just one day, I wonder how far they would stretch? From St. Louis to Chicago? To New York?

Not too long ago, I took part in a closing communion service at an ecumenical retreat center in the mountains of Wyoming, about an hour from the Grand Tetons. I looked down as folks went by and realized that I could recognize them by their shoes — work boots, cowboy boots, sandals, running shoes. The shoes of each individual were special — connecting them to their work and to the passions in their lives. The cowboy boots belonged to the old wrangler who selected and cared for the horses on the ranch — China, Dusty, El Salvador. The work boots, scuffed and muddy, were on the handyman who fixed the barbed-wire fences, the patched-together plumbing, the Massey Ferguson. The artist who spent little time among the rocks and scrub, content to wander from studio to lunch, wore Birkenstocks. A high school girl who ran the mountain roads in the thin, cool air of the morning bore Reeboks.

A friend of mine, who is a nun, gave me a photograph of a dark-skinned pair of dusty feet in sandals, which I have kept on my desk for many years. It is a precious image to me. For the photo of those sandals, and those dusty feet, represents not only Christ, who walked so many miles to care for others, but each and every one of us who is called to be healing people. We are called to serve God and humankind, using the unique wisdom, knowledge, and gifts we have each been given. Our feet — and our hands, hearts, and heads — are needed by God in the work of healing in the world. "It takes a village," said Hillary Rodham Clinton. "It takes a lot of shoes," I say.

May God bless your shoes and the healing work they carry you to do, today and always. Blessings as you continue your marvelous work of healing in the community, and in God's world.

prayers

While these prayers are written from a Christian perspective and a primarily Christian cultural context, they can be adapted for use with people of differing faiths. I have sometimes chosen to end a prayer in a traditional Christian way, namely, "In Jesus' name." In other cases, I have ended prayers in a more inclusive manner, such as, "We pray in your precious name" or "I pray in your name, O God, who is greater than all." The reader is encouraged to adapt these prayers to be sensitive to the faith perspective of those with whom or for whom one is praying.

23

Prayer for Healing

Healing can happen in one of three ways: first, through the healing that the body does naturally, such as when a person has a cold; second, through medical intervention, such as through the administration of antibiotics or through a surgical procedure; and third and most finally, through the process of dying.

This prayer was written with the understanding that God can bless and heal us in a number of ways, and so it is dedicated to those of us (all of us!) who are praying for God's healing presence in our lives.

Loving and tender God, touch my heart with hope, touch my mind with clarity, touch my soul with peace, and touch my body with the warmth of your healing presence.

Grant me courage to face the future, insight to understand life's trials, wisdom to discern how I can touch the lives of others, and comfort of people who care about me as I reach for your loving hands. In Jesus' name, Amen.

24

Prayer of Blessing for Healers

This prayer was written for those who work in hospitals, clinics, and in other health-care settings. It can be used as part of a "Health Care Sunday" in a church, as an opening devotion for a meeting in a hospital, or for private meditation.

Healing God, bless the healers in this place, and throughout your world. Lead us all to greater understanding of your love and purpose for all Creation. Help those who are called as healers to embrace their roles as leaders in the community, calling others into fullness of life.

Loving God, bless the healers, who carry the mantle of responsibility for knowledge of body, mind, and spirit, and knowledge of your saving grace. Grant them power to change lives — beginning with their own. Help them to forge paths to the healing waters, where renewal and comfort are found.

Caring God, bless the healers, who bear the strain of worry for those who are afflicted with pain and sorrow. You have promised to all who are heavy-laden a yoke which is easy and a burden which is light. We know that you bear the weight of the world, but we also know that the healers who walk alongside those who suffer are not untouched by their trouble.

Hopeful God, bless the healers, who give their lives in service of others. Bless them as they point toward wholeness, and peace, and hope. Bless them as they search for answers to life's questions. Bless them as they pray and minister unto others.

Bless them as they walk in their own sorrow and pain.

Living God, bless the healers. And bless all those with whom the healers live, and work, and have their being. We pray in your precious name. Amen.

25

Prayer of Blessing for Healers in the Church

This prayer was written as a blessing for parish nurses in the church, but can be adapted as a blessing for others doing health ministries as well.

Generous and empathetic God, bless these parish nurses whom you have called as your disciples, so that they may touch and bless all those among whom they minister. Guide them by the wisdom of your Holy Spirit, so they may be empowered to go where they are most needed. May they be filled with courage, to speak the truth in love and to act boldly on behalf of those who are in need of healing and understanding.

Touch these nurses, who are your faithful servants, with tender comfort as they walk with those in pain and fear, so that they may serve as a reminder of your eternal compassion. When they are weary, hold each of them gently in your loving arms and sing to them songs of hope and refreshment. Let each of them sing praises daily to you for your faithfulness and loving kindness to all Creation.

Let them never give in to cynicism or despair, but help them always to feel your sustaining presence, calling them on. Bless their ministry as nurses, this day, and always, we pray in Jesus' name. Amen.

26

Prayer for Renewal

Health-care professionals and clergy often begin their careers with a burning desire to help others. The need for help by others, however, is absolutely unlimited, and no human being can meet everyone's needs. Sometimes people in such professions become worn-out and feel as though there will be no end to the demands. When this occurs, it is necessary to step back, take a breath, and look for sources of renewal.

It's hard to get out of this lonely rut — I've been here for so long! Help me listen for the winds of your Spirit blowing change, bringing the cooling rains of renewal and the bright dawn of hope.

Help me to relax and draw a deep draught of your refreshing presence. Help me to see something new today and be open to those who surround me. Surely you, in your infinite variety of design and thought, can show me a path through this unchanging wilderness. Train my eyes on the mountains, a river, an oasis, a spring, where I may drink and find hope for my soul.

Then, O God, help me journey toward healing of body, soul, and mind, so that I may come through the valley of the shadow of doubt and fear, for you are with me. When I am in pain, let me hold fast to your rod and your staff, that they might uphold me, direct me, and comfort me, as you lead me according to your purposes and my heartfelt longings and abilities.

This I pray in your name, O God who is greater than all. Amen.

27

Prayer of Preparation

This prayer is a morning prayer for those who face patients and parishioners in need of healing and hope.

> *Guide my feet today, O God of wisdom and strength. Guide my hands as I reach out to care skillfully for others who have put their trust in me. Even more, gentle healer, guide my heart, so that I may be open to your presence and the needs of your people bringing their fears and pain.*
>
> *Forgive me for any harm I may unintentionally cause this day, and help me to forgive myself for not being all things to all people. And at the end of the day, help me to release each person into your compassionate care, for ultimately, I am only an instrument of your healing. I pray in your Precious Name, Amen.*

28

Prayer for a Healer Who is Overwhelmed

Society expects its doctors to be gods and its ministers to be infallible. They expect healers to be all things to all people, at all times of the day and night. This prayer is for a healer who finds herself/himself overwhelmed. Who among us has not been there?

Too much, O God! Too much! Even Jesus, who could heal with a word, or the touch of his hand, got into a boat to escape. Even he felt, at times, overwhelmed by the needs of the poor, the hungry, the suffering, and the sorrowing. Help me, O God!

Help me not to turn away in self-defense, but help me to turn people toward other sources of healing, including the healing power of a natural death, when all other paths have ended. Give me the courage to stay with the dying.

Remind me of my roots in you, as healer and guide to the afflicted. Heal and guide me, as well, O God, for I also am in need of the touch of your gentle and comforting Spirit.

Please encourage me — the fields are white unto harvest with work to be done, but I cannot harvest every day. Send relief: Send workers out into the field to labor with me. Repair the breaches in community that place such a heavy burden on all the healers.

Help me to remember that, ultimately, you are the source of all healing.

An antibiotic only stops the bacteria from spreading so that the body can win. A scalpel can remove a growth, but then the body must heal itself. A clergy can bring a word of hope, but you are the One who opens hearts. As a healer, I can make a contribution; then I must leave the rest to you. And then I can rest in you.

Heal my weary bones and spirit, heal my weary heart. I can't see you! Too many people suffer — too many people die. Too few people take care of themselves — too few people live as they should. I am tired of hearing their stories. Do you feel like that, too?

Relieve me from being God, my God. Remind me again how to minister and be ministered to as a sacred healer of your beloved people. In Jesus' name, Amen.

29

Prayer for the Patients

This small prayer is for the patients of doctors and chaplains, who are being remembered in prayer by their families and friends, by their pastors and their faith communities. A health-care setting can be a sacred place where people experience the range of human emotion and come to know God's loving care as they experience the presence of others who care about them.

Whispering God, whose still, small voice can be heard in the quiet of the night, in the break of dawn, and at the close of the day, let your loving Spirit surround each of the patients coming to, in, and going from this place, with healing and hope. May they be strengthened and helped by all with whom they have contact.

May the treatment of each person in this place be careful, wise, and compassionate. May they be inspired to reach for their own healing in partnership with those who are treating and caring for them. May they feel safe and valued, and may they embrace the fullness of your healing love.

Keep them from harm and fear, and guide the work of each one with whom they have contact this day. May their journeys of healing be blessed, and may they each know the comfort of spiritual sustenance. Help each one to a place of wholeness, we pray, in your Holy Name. Amen.

30

Prayer for the Emergency Department

An emergency room is a place of refuge for people who are in immediate need of healing. Often they are terribly frightened, as are their loved ones. The emergency room is also the last refuge for the uninsured; it must by law treat the uninsured, who often have no access to primary care elsewhere. Working toward universal health-care coverage should be a priority of all faith communities.

> *Loving God, through these doors walk (or are carried or wheeled in with haste) the injured, the wounded, the dying, the suffering, the sorrowing, and the frightened. No one comes through these doors without cause, though some may be drawn to human contact from aching loneliness or are trying to slip into the waiting area to warm themselves. The emergency room, like Jesus, seems to attract many different people at all hours of the day and night. For many who need medical attention in this country, the health care found beyond these sacred doors is their only resort.*
>
> *Gracious One, touch the hearts of the overworked clerks, orderlies, technicians, nurses, and doctors who care for those who have entrusted their very lives to the mercy and skill of those in this emergency room this day, this evening, in the middle of the night. Bless the babies that come through here, the children, the parents, and the aging. Bless those who are caught in the middle — the insured and the uninsured, who wait and still wait, and who pray for recovery and for compassion.*

Help those who care for them to be courageous and patient, insightful and wise, persistent and comforting. We remember that you have called each of us to bring healing to the world. We pray for those working in all places of such brokenness and hope, and for those who enter, broken and hopeful. This we pray in the name of Jesus, who longs to bring healing and hope to all. Amen.

31

Prayer for the Surgical Suites

To many people, the operating rooms are the inner sanctuary of a hospital — the Holy of Holies, where the most sacred work is done. The inner space of the body is invasively entered during surgery, and those who participate in this ritual have a moral and sacred duty to do no harm, to prevent further harm, and to actively promote the welfare of the patient. This prayer is for that sacred place, for the remarkable people who toil there, and for the patients who enter with hope and trepidation.

> *God of all mystery, let your Holy Presence fill these surgical suites with healing light. Grant your strength to all those who work here, and guide their thoughts, words, and actions, so that together, their hands may restore wholeness to all who seek healing in this place. Unfold the mysteries of the body in layers before them, and show them pathways to guide their instruments. When they find they are unable to see, but only able to feel or sense, be their constant guide.*
>
> *God of all comfort, be closer than breath to all those who enter here for a surgical procedure this day. Help them to hear words of encouragement and hope, no matter what their condition. We know that you are always with us, to show our spirits a way through all challenges that lie before us. Keep all who pass this way today in your loving arms, and hold them as they go forth. We thank you for the healing instincts that you have placed in each of our bodies, which seek to knit us back to wholeness.*

God of all strength, we pray that you would be with those who wait, who anxiously await word of the condition of their loved ones who are undergoing surgery. We pray for those who wait for a word of hope, a word of truth, a word of solace. Lift them up and carry them through this day and through the days ahead as they pray for and care for their loved ones.

God of the universe, we pray for those who will come into this place after the surgeries are over. Bless those who will clean these surgical suites and prepare these doors to receive others tomorrow, that their work be done as a sacred task as well.

All these things we pray in your sacred name. Amen.

32

Prayer for the Health of the Congregation — I

Most congregations pray regularly for the sick. Prayer for the sick is important and a biblical injunction. It should be part of the life of a worshiping community.

A theology of wholeness and wellness, however, would also include a word of thanksgiving and support for those who are healthy and who are seeking to be good stewards of the blessings of God's earth through guardianship of clean water, air, good food, as well as through guardianship of their bodies as they exercise and celebrate life.

> *Teach us, O God, how to walk in paths of wholeness and hope. Help us to care for those among us who are sick, and to challenge those who are well to embrace the fullness and vigor of life that you bring.*
>
> *Let those who are lonely or sorrowing be comforted and called back into community. Let those who are depressed or suffering from mental anguish be helped through compassionate care and support. Let those who are facing illness of body be encouraged and assisted as they seek to recover or be released from their pain. Let those who are healthy celebrate with joy. Let those of us who are able honor your creation through thankful enjoyment of nutritious food, clean air and water, and vigorous exercise, rejoicing in the splendid variety of your creation.*
>
> *Help us to be a healthy and healing congregation, O God, as place where all are free to live fully in body, mind, and spirit. This we pray in your precious name. Amen.*

33

Prayer for the Health of the Congregation — II

This prayer lifts up health in our global context.

> *Compassionate God, we pray for those in fear:*
> ~ *those in fear of the personal change and transformation to which you call us;*
> ~ *those in fear of violence and persecution by individuals and political systems seeking domination and control of others;*
> ~ *those in fear of the unknown circumstances that lie ahead of them, their families, and their communities.*
> *God, in your mercy, hear our prayer.*
>
> *Healing God, we pray for those in pain:*
> ~ *those in pain from grief and loss of loved ones held dear;*
> ~ *those in physical or mental pain from illness or infirmity;*
> ~ *those in pain from the place in which they find themselves in community, from hunger or isolation.*
> *God, in your mercy, hear our prayer.*
>
> *Merciful God, we pray for the stubborn:*
> ~ *that you would turn their hearts to your ways of wholeness and peace;*
> ~ *that you would fill them with courage to follow in your paths of wisdom and righteousness;*
> ~ *that you would open their minds to the possibilities for new*

life that surrounds them in your love;
God, in your mercy, hear our prayer.

Gracious and eternal God, we pray for the fearful, pain-filled stubborn places in which we all find ourselves. Help us to embrace your paths of healing and well-being and to release our fears, our pain, and our stubbornness to you. Teach us joy, hope, and courage so that we may bring joy, hope, and courage to others in your name.

We pray for peace and wholeness in the churches and among people of other faiths throughout the world, that your ways would be our ways.

God, in your mercy, hear our prayer.

34

A Prayer for Health During the Holiday Season

On average, people living in Canada and the United States gain just one pound (net) during the holiday season (that's just Thanksgiving-Christmas), but those pounds add up over the years! Advent is the time to mentally and spiritually plan for healthy physical habits over the winter months.

Loving and intimate God, thank you for these days of harvest and homecoming that lead us into the holy days of remembering your presence with us. As we remember the years gone by, we give thanks for loved ones who have gone before, who nurtured us with hugs and hot chocolate, kisses and cookies. Help us to dwell on the hugs and kisses, and to pass those on to our loved ones.

We remember the joy of celebrating Holy Days and holidays with food, and we long for things to be special. Help us to remember that as your people, we are already special in your accepting eyes, much more than any meal we could prepare. Fill our emptiness — the spiritual hunger, loneliness, and insecurity that we feel. Help us see that we are loved for who we are, not for what we cook or bake for others. Help us to celebrate our precious bodies and to care for them with nourishing and health-giving food.

Generous and encouraging God, show us how to meditate on your sacred and perfect nature, and not get caught by the seductive promises of earthly perfection that beckon from magazine headlines. Help us not to fall into the trap of believing that "this year we will do it right." Everything is already right when we are right with you.

And finally, eternal God of summer, fall, winter, and spring, empower us to move our bodies each day in response to your love, as we run joyfully into the future you have prepared for us. In your loving name we pray, Amen.

35

Prayer for the Aging

The majority of time and resources of most healers is spent helping the elderly. We are all aging; this prayer is for those who are currently elderly, and for us all.

Eternal God, we give you thanks for the immortal spirit wrapped within each human body. From fragile birth to robust youth to years of weakening frame, you are our strength and guide. You are the source of all that was, and is, and is to be.

Take from us the fear of aging. Help us to know that we will not die all deaths but only one. Reveal to us your Spirit, greater than uncertainty and larger than loss. Open our minds, hearts, and spirits to new paths.

If we should be afflicted with chronic illness that threatens to eclipse our independence, help us to settle into you for comfort and nurture. Teach us to trust you, merciful God, and help us to be open to your ways. As embodied spirits of your creation, even the young have but a brief span remaining on earth. You, who are from everlasting to everlasting, the Wisdom of the Ages, the source of every blessing, can show us the power of opening ourselves to spiritual seasons of growth. Soften our fears — of pain, loss, grief, or separation from all that we love. Comfort us with the assurance that you are capable and willing of good beyond that which we know.

Help us to live each day in fullness of life — to enjoy friends and family, eat well, exercise, sleep, work, play, and celebrate.

If disease or injury should somehow sideline us before our spirits return to you, remind us daily of our infinite worth. And when our time has come to leave this embodied company, help our spirits to dance into death, embraced by you and all the saints who have gone before our time.

Thank you now for each precious day of life in which to smell the rain and feel the wind. What a remarkable journey our spirits are on! Surely goodness and mercy shall follow us all the days of our lives, and we shall dwell in the house of the Lord forever!

36

Prayer for Seniors in Residential Care

At any given time, about 5 percent of the senior population in America lives in residential care. It is a time that can be difficult or made easier by compassionate healers.

Loving God, you lead us down paths that surprise us, and you help us all the days of our lives. We pray this day for those who are in residential care, that you may surround them with a sense of home. Let those who provide care to them be compassionate, let those who befriend them be gentle, and let those who meet them be kind.

Guard them, O God, from harm. Heal their bodies and spirits, whether through recovery of their former abilities, through the acceptance and embrace of the present reality, or through the final relief of release brought through a peaceful death.

We pray for those whose loved ones live in residential care. Grant them the ability to visit often, to advocate well, to be attentive, and to sustain their care and devotion through all the days that lie ahead.

When you ask each one of us to depart this life, bring joy in the morning. Until that day, bring humor and light. We pray in the name of the One who is the Light of the World. In Jesus' name, Amen.

37

Prayer for Homebound Seniors

This prayer, which is written for use by individuals or groups praying for homebound seniors as a group, may be adapted as a prayer for an individual who is homebound.

Loving God, we lift up to you in prayer this day those who are homebound and ask that you bless them with purpose and hope. Help them to know connection beyond their own walls, and grant the ability to fulfill all those tasks to which you are calling them.

Heal them of fear and loneliness, and walk with them through the infirmities that are challenging them. Help them to reach out to others when they need support, and to offer their own prayers and compassion when needed by others. You call us all to responsibility, Lord. Remind us all that in Christ we are one Body, and that each has a part to play.

We pray for the family members and friends of the homebound and ask that you help them as they seek to be a support. Help them to do what they can, to ask for help when they need it, and to know when to go home.

Finally, God, we ask for your spiritual blessing upon the homebound that they may know your ever-dawning presence, shining even brighter with clarity and understanding. May their homebound sojourn be a home-bound journey, leading ever nearer to you. This we pray in Jesus' name, Amen.

38

Prayer for Someone Facing Surgery

A patient must relinquish control of their body in order to undergo surgery, and the thought of someone cutting into one's body is fearsome. We know that patients are greatly affected by their attitude going into surgery, and we are learning that they are able to perceive more while under anesthesia than we earlier thought possible. This prayer for guidance is for all who are involved in this sacred process of opening the body for healing.

> *God who surrounds us, who goes before and behind us, who knows us all within and without, go with (NAME) as she/he prepares for surgery. Go before him/her and help him/her to rest on the ocean of your gentle presence. Help him/her to be calm and focused, to stay relaxed and strong throughout the surgery, and then to rally for a steady recovery. Stay very near.*
>
> *Guide the hands, minds, and hearts of the healers performing the surgery and surrounding him/her with prayer and support. Show the healing team the best way into and around the sacred realm of (NAME's) body, and help them to support his/her mind and spirit all through this procedure and during the recovery. Surround all those in the operating suite this day with a spirit of patience and courage as their hands work quickly and well within your healing work.*
>
> *Help (NAME) to remember that there is nowhere we can go from your presence — neither life nor death nor anything else in all creation can separate us from the love of God.*

Be with those who watch and wait, help them as they pray for (NAME), and grant them all strength and hope, this day and in the days ahead.

We pray in your loving and holy name. Amen.

39

Prayer for Someone Who has Received a Serious Diagnosis

It's a frightening moment. The test results show that the diagnosis is serious. Yet each person's health, body, and attitude are different. So what comes next?

God of the unknown future, we thank you that your Spirit goes before us in all circumstances, and your abiding love will not let us go. Be with (NAME) as she/he begins a journey through understanding and coping with this illness. May all that she/he does and all that the medical, nursing, and faith communities around her/him do be supportive of wholeness and fullness of life.

We pray that you would bring clarity of understanding to all who are treating (NAME) for this illness, and that you would bring him/her peace and hope. We pray that she/he would be spared all undue suffering, and that her/his friends, family, and neighbors would rally around him/her to provide comfort and support.

We pray that you would encourage and strengthen (NAME) and her/his family so that no stone is left unturned in the search for a way through this illness with dignity and compassion.

Where there is fear, bring comfort; where there is pain, bring relief; where there is sadness, bring solace. Loving God, where there is loneliness, bring the fellowship of family, friends, and the communion of saints.

How fragile are our bodies, O God! Yet how strong are our

spirits! You know and love us and will not let us go, and your strength and courage are eternal. We thank you for your presence with (NAME) and with us all. In Jesus' name we pray, Amen.

40

Prayer for Someone Who has Suffered an Accident

In an instant, a life can be transformed through an accident. The injured one, and his or her family members and friends, try to make sense of and find meaning in the traumatic event. They also experience great anxiety as they seek to understand the extent and full effect of injuries. Often these processes are occurring at the same time.

> *Dear God,*
>
> *We are angry and afraid that this accident has happened. We know that you did not cause it and that there is no higher purpose within the accident itself. It is a terrible situation!*
>
> *Help us to remember that when one of your people suffers, you suffer as well. You long to comfort and console each one of us and lead us through the valley of the shadow of death.*
>
> *Be with (NAME), and help him/her through this valley. As spiritual beings in a human frame, we need the strength of your Spirit to bring courage and hope. Show (NAME) a path to wholeness and peace.*
>
> *We ask that you would surround us all with your peace, helping us to know that you will never leave us or forsake us. We give thanks that you will stay with (NAME) both day and night, keeping a constant vigil and granting him/her strength.*
>
> *Guide the work of each healer helping (NAME) and grant each one insight into the best course of treatment. Loving God, guide (NAME's) thoughts so that he/she may find a way through this trauma to newness of life. Wrap your tender*

arms around her/him and keep her/him close. This we pray
in your precious name, Amen.

Prayer for Someone Who has Suffered an Accident

41

Prayer for a Runaway

Every day over a million runaway and homeless youth live on the streets of America. Some are running from serious problems at home while others are living with mental illness. This prayer is for the family and the runaway.

Precious Savior,
Surely you remember the panic that your parents expressed
when you were in the temple and they left Jerusalem, thinking
you were with them. Certainly you remember the pain in your
mother's eyes as they took you away to be crucified. We know
that you understand the pain and grief of the family we lift up
before you this day. We pray for them, dear Savior, and ask you
to surround each one of them with your compassionate arms.

Watch over (NAME), who has chosen to leave his/her home
at this time. Help him/her to feel your presence near and to
find safety, hope, and healing soon. Watch over her/his parent(s)
in the coming days, and help them to trust that there will be
a way through this terrifying time of fear and guilt, despair
and worry.

Grant them your strength, for you have known the worst
that the world can offer, and still you discovered ways to be
friend and guide. You did not turn your back on your people
but simply said, "Abba, forgive them, for they know not what
they do."

Grant this family hope, courage, and peace. Help each of
them to know that there is nothing — neither life, nor death,

nor things present, nor things to come, nor heights, nor depths, nor angels, nor principalities, nor anything else in all Creation — that can separate us from the love of God in Christ Jesus. It is in your compassionate name of wisdom and mercy that we pray. Amen.

42

Prayer for Someone in Prison

Fear. Loneliness. Isolation. Worry about loved ones at home. Shame. Humiliation. Financial concerns. Anger. Rage. So many emotions flood a person who has been imprisoned. There are many roles that healers can play to assist those in prison, from serving as chaplains, nurses, doctors, or guides for the journey back home.

Growing numbers of the incarcerated are women, reflected here in the use of the female pronoun. Pronouns should be changed as appropriate.

> *Loving God, please help (NAME), who has been imprisoned, and help her to know that we have not forgotten her. Even more importantly, help her to know that you will never leave or forsake her. Help her to know that we will surround her and her loved ones with help and care. Help her to know that we will visit her and stay in touch with her while she is in prison. And help her to know that we will help her when she comes home.*
>
> *Open the gates of the prison in her heart and mind, O God, and lead her into freedom and newness of life. Help her to claim her infinite worth and value to you, and to others in Creation. Help her to believe in herself and in the possibilities for change.*
>
> *Keep her safe, O God, and occupy her mind so that the time in prison will not weigh too heavily on her. Help her to grow nearer to your Holy Presence and to seek the good in others.*
>
> *Loving God, you know the guilt and innocence of us all.*

No one is all good. No one is all bad. We know that none can stand blameless before you. Turn all hearts to you, God of wisdom and justice, and help us all to find a way through the wilderness that leads to fullness of life for all people. This we pray in Jesus' name, Amen.

Prayer for Someone in Prison

43

Prayer for the Loss of a Loved One

For some, death comes as a shock, for some as a tragedy, and for others as a blessed release from protracted suffering. Each death is personal, as is each response to that person's death, depending on the nature of the relationship between the loved ones and the circumstances surrounding the death. Yet there are some commonalities when a death occurs — realization of the finality of the spiritual transition of bodily death, some regrets for words that were left unspoken and deeds that were left undone, and gratitude for that person's life, even when the relationship had been rocky.

> *Sheltering God, hold (NAME) close as she/he grieves the loss of her/his beloved (relationship/name). This severing of earthly ties feels final, yet we know that the life of the spirit is eternal. We mourn the death of (NAME), whose bodily life on earth has ended, but whose spirit will live on in the memories of all those who knew and loved her/him. May he/she rest in peace, for we know that for him/her, all fear and pain is over. We ask you to release his/her loved ones from regrets, and keep them close to all that was good about (NAME).*
>
> *When sorrow overtakes them, surround them with strength. Help them grieve and remember. Help them take care of themselves, and give themselves time to recover but never to forget. Send them friends who will encourage them and be with them in the hours of heavy sorrow. Help them lean on you for support, for you have suffered many losses in this world and are acquainted with grief.*

All these things we pray in the name of your beloved and eternal Son, Jesus the Christ. Amen.

44

Prayer for the Loss of a Child

"Absolom — my son! My son!" cried David, King of all Israel. He wept, he tore his clothes, he put on sackcloth and ashes, yet despite his prayers, his beloved son died. Jesus' mother, Mary, stood at the foot of the cross as he suffered a criminal's death of crucifixion. She would not leave him, even unto death.

Loving God, you know that (NAMES) did everything possible to save their child and would not leave him/her, even unto death. Be with them now as they face the rest of their earthly life without their precious child. Hold them gently in your compassionate arms and comfort them, even as you gently hold the spirit of their beloved son/daughter and comfort him/her for all eternity. We thank you that for their child, all suffering is past and he/she is truly free from pain and fear.

Please help them to know that there is nowhere we can go from your presence — neither life, nor death, nor height, nor depths, nor things present, nor things to come, nor angels, nor principalities, nor anything else in all creation can separate us from the love of God in Christ Jesus our Lord. Please help this family to know that their precious one will never again be afraid, lonely, or distressed, as he/she is being held by you, whose name is Love. And let your strong arms hold them all as they grieve until they are once again reunited in your kingdom which has no end. Blessing and honor, glory and power be unto you, O Lord, Jesus Christ. Amen and amen.

45

Prayer for the Family of an Organ Donor

For those who are faced with the difficult task of acknowledging the sudden death of a loved one, the option of donating organs (if that would have been the deceased's choice) provides hope for at least a small portion of good to have come out of a tragic and unchangeable situation.

> *Dear God,*
>
> *We pray for the family of (NAME), who has agreed to the donation of his/her organs. They do this believing that this act would be in accordance with (NAME's) wishes, so that some good may come from this terrible loss.*
>
> *Bless the process of transplanting all organs and tissue that may be used. May each procedure be successful and without complications. We pray that you would grant new hope to the recipient(s) and help them to renew their strength.*
>
> *Comfort and encourage this family that they may hold on to the assurance that they have done all they could to add to the infinite value of the life of their beloved (NAME).*
>
> *May each recipient of these organs and each of their families, who thankfully and gratefully receive these precious gifts, always remember the life of the one who has died. May they also remember the compassionate act of this family, who has chosen to share life with others.*
>
> *All these things we pray in your Holy Name. Amen.*

46

Prayer for the Family of an Organ/Tissue Recipient

The joy of receiving an organ for the family of someone who has been waiting is always tempered to some degree by the empathetic thought that someone else has lost a loved one. This prayer tries to acknowledge both of these realities.

Loving God, we gratefully acknowledge this life-sustaining act of organ/tissue donation, freely given because of one whose life has been tragically cut short. We ask your comfort and blessing upon the deceased's family, that you would be with them in the coming days. Help them to know how grateful we are that (NAME) has received this inestimable gift, and how thankful we are to them for having made this decision to share a vital part of their loved one's life.

We pray that this organ/this tissue will be successfully integrated into the body of (NAME) and that she/he may now be rapidly healed and renewed. We thank you that for him/her, the waiting for an organ/tissue transplant is over. We know it has been a long, painful, and frightening journey. Bless and sustain us all, as we seek each day to do your will in all things, through Christ, our Savior. Amen.

47

Prayer for Someone Facing Death

The hardest part of life is death — letting go of our loved ones and facing our own mortality. It is not an option. For some, death is a release; for others, a terrible crossing. This prayer is for all who are facing death.

Comfort, comfort, O God, this your suffering one, who leans on you now for guidance and hope. You call us from the unrecoverable space we know as death, and from there you promise something more.

We knew no suffering before our earthly days, and we thank you that for (NAME), all pain and sorrow will soon be past. The dying journey is solitary and unsearchable, and we do not fully know or comprehend its truths. Help us, eternal and everlasting God.

Our world is a richness of color and timbre, texture and fragrance, a sonorous banquet for body, mind, and spirit. We worry that without our bodily senses there will be a blank palette. We worry about those we leave behind. We want to help them, hold them, and love them more. We will.

Please help us hold on to hope, to memories, to wisdom gained from our love. And help us let go of pain, of fear, of despair, of sorrow — and to reach out for your loving presence.

Yea, even though we walk through the valley of the shadow of death, we fear no evil, for you are ever, always, with us. Fill us with your peace and your transcendent, life-transforming Spirit. Bless and keep (NAME), your precious one, and help him/her through this silent valley into the splendor of your healing presence. In Jesus' name, Amen.

48

Prayer for Someone Who is Depressed

According to the National Mental Health Association, depression affects over nineteen million Americans each year. Adolescents and children can also experience clinical depression. There is help — through the support of families, friends, the medical community, and the faith community. NAMI (The National Alliance for the Mentally Ill) has more information at 1-800-950-NAMI (6264) or on their Web site at *www.nami.org*.

> *Out of the depths, O God, we cry to you! God, hear the groan of this your beloved, who is caught in the grips of despair and desolation. How many people have walked through these shadows, yet it feels to each that they bear alone the growing weight of the world.*
>
> *Be with (NAME), O God. Bless him/her and keep him/her in your loving care. We know that the Spirit prays for us in our weakness and intercedes for us according to your holy will. Lift up (NAME) and lighten his/her path — through medication, therapy, support of family and/or friends. We know that your compassion is towards all — your love knows no bounds. We believe in faith that, despite our feelings to the contrary at times, you will never leave us or forsake us.*
>
> *Guard the spirit and strength of this, your precious one, and help us all to lend our support in ways that bring hope.*
>
> *All these things we pray in the name of Jesus, the Christ. Amen.*

49

Prayer for the "Dark Night of the Soul"

Many health-care providers and clergy go through a "dark night of the soul" on their spiritual journey. It is a time of deep spiritual growth, but it can be frightening and isolating. Here is a prayer to console you during those hours.

I thank you, O God, that there is nowhere I can go from your presence. Neither life, nor death, nor anything else in all Creation can separate your love from me, or me from the shelter of your strengthening arms.

Hide me in your darkness, O God, for there are no shadows in you. Illuminate my paths, and help me see where I am going. Save me from the drudgery of eternal sameness. Help me to listen for your voice and to answer when you call.

It is night in my soul, but with you, the night is the same as day. Grant water and new surprises for my thirsty soul, food and new directions for my hungry spirit, and when the day is done, blessed rest for my body and mind. Amen.

50

Prayer for Work

In their book, *The Two-Income Trap: Why Middle-Class Mothers and Fathers are Going Broke,* authors Elizabeth Warren and Amelia Warren Tyagi project that by the end of the decade, more families will declare bankruptcy each year than are diagnosed during that time with cancer.[1] With many jobs moving abroad and companies downsizing to avoid the rising costs of health-care coverage, you may wish to offer this "Prayer for Work" as part of a worship experience or gathering in your faith community.

> *God of eternity, who created the world in joyful splendor and then rested, secure in the knowledge that there would be more work to come, we pray that you would surround your faithful servants, who have been seeking to serve you with all their hearts, and all their minds, and all their souls, and all their strength. Some are afraid that they might lose their jobs; others fear that they might fall ill and be unable to perform their tasks, while some of your people worry that their work is in vain.*
>
> *What is humankind, O God, that you are mindful of us? How do you notice our pains and our fears? How do you comfort? How do you heal?*
>
> *Salve the wounds of fear facing your people, O God, and show each of us a way through this desert of uncertainty, to springs of hope ahead. We remember our Savior, Jesus the Christ, who was born in a manger, and faced the challenges of faithfulness in the midst of ambiguity. Like Jesus, we are*

tempted by the one who said that to be free we must be rich in worldly things.

Help us to remember that all things work together for good for those who love God, who are called according to God's purposes. Help us to remember that you know what we need, that you know when we lie down, and when we rise up, when we go out, and when we come in. Help us not to be anxious but to trust that you will keep us from this day forth, and forevermore. Help us to seek you in all that we do for our work so that our work may be that of helping to bring about your Realm on earth.

This we pray in the name of Jesus, who taught us to trust in you. Amen.

51

Prayer for Someone Who is Moving

Moving is a significant stressor on a person's health, particularly when combined with other changes such as friendships, work responsibilities, or schools. A church community often can help by providing meals, muscles, and prayers.

> *Widen our world, O God, and smooth the paths for (NAMES), who are moving from our midst. Go before them to open the hearts of those who will call them colleagues, neighbors, and friends. Soften the hearts of those who will help them on their journey, prepare a path before them, and show them your ways to newness of life. Bless their new home, their new workplace(s), their new congregation, and their new community.*

If there are children in the family who are also moving:

> *We ask a special blessing upon their children, that you might help them know all will be well. Lead them to new friends and teachers who will enfold them in welcome.*
>
> *Just as Abraham and Sarah left on a promise and found great blessing, may this family find new hope and blessing on their journey and at the journey's end.*
>
> *We pray in Jesus' name. Amen.*

52

Prayer for Someone Who Cannot Sleep

Within the Islamic faith, there is a tradition of the ninety-nine names of God. A helpful spiritual discipline in the middle of a sleepless night may be to think of the names for God that have special meaning for you. Some of the names for God in the Christian faith include: Wonderful, Holy One, Redeemer, Savior, Merciful One, Healer, Counselor, Father, Mother, Everlasting God, and the Prince of Peace, among many others. The hymn text by Bryan Wren, "Bring Many Names," may bring soothing thoughts to one who is wrestling with wakefulness. Others find great peace in saying the Rosary or other familiar prayers.

> *Thank you, O Lord, for this time to meditate upon you and your wondrous works. As I breathe, I number your precious names.* (Begin to think about the many ways God can be named, and meditate upon each of the names.)
>
> *I breathe in your goodness....* (Concentrate on your breathing, but do not hold your breath. Relax and enjoy the rhythmic patterns of your breathing.)
>
> *If this doesn't work, get up and read the Bible. Choose a Bible verse on which to meditate, such as "God gives sleep to his beloved" (Psalm 127:2b). Reading the Bible will eventually put you to sleep. (Of course, this works with most other books as well.)*

53

Prayer at the Birth of a Child

Sometimes the birth of a child is a greatly anticipated event in the life of a
mother or family. At other times, an unplanned pregnancy and childbirth is
no less of a miracle, but worrisome for the mother or parents. Given that
nearly half of all pregnancies in developed countries are unplanned, healers
should allow room for ambiguity in a prayer at the birth of a child.

> *Miraculous God, we give you thanks and praise for the*
> *birth of this wonderful child, a new creation in your world.*
> *Called and formed by you before he/she was born, you have a*
> *plan for this child, to give him/her a future and a hope.*
>
> *Bless (NAME[S]), and be to her/them a source of inspira-*
> *tion, guidance, comfort, and assurance as she/they seek(s) to*
> *nurture and raise this child. Help her/them to know that*
> *she/they is/are not alone, and that, as a loving God, you will*
> *never leave nor forsake them. Help her/them to remember*
> *that there are no perfect parents, but that love casts out fear.*
>
> *Bless this child, that she/he might find a special place in*
> *your world, and that she/he might know sheltering love and*
> *care all the days of his/her life. Let him/her find joy in learning*
> *and growing, and welcome in a loving community. Grant to*
> *him/her health and longevity, happiness and peace.*
>
> *All these things we pray in your Holy Name, Amen.*

54

Prayer for Someone Facing Infertility

When someone is infertile, it seems the whole world is filled with pregnancies and babies. Infertility can make a woman and/or man feel incompetent and broken. The feeling of powerlessness often leads people to invest great resources in technologies that sometimes, but not always, lead to success. It is a painful, trying dilemma.

> *Creator God, how difficult it is for a woman and man who long to create new life and share their love with a child, when they are facing infertility! How painful it is to go through Christmas each year, celebrating the birth of a baby to one who was not expecting such an event in her life! How hard it is to go through Mother's Day year after year, when women with children seem to be everywhere, highly honored and valued.*
>
> *Be with this couple, O God, and help them to know that they are precious and good. Help them as they go through medical interventions to assist them in starting a family. We pray that you would strengthen their spirits (and their relationship with each other) so that they may not become disheartened and isolated. Help them to take good care of themselves so that they may only pursue those paths to childbirth that bring hope and peace, and not place them in harm's way.*
>
> *God of wisdom and understanding, illumine the paths of their journey, that it may be one filled with love. Grant them wisdom and understanding, hope and courage as they seek to provide love and care to children of their own. Through Christ our Redeemer we pray. Amen.*

55

Prayer for Someone Waiting to Adopt a Child

The waiting to adopt does not involve the physical stress of pregnancies, but there are many other similarities. This prayer acknowledges the reality of the child soon to arrive and the feelings — stress, anxiety, glory — that surround the waiting parent(s).

Many single parents now adopt, so pronouns should be changed as is appropriate.

> *Loving God, you gather your children from north and south, east and west. How you tend carefully for each of your loved ones!*
>
> *Be with (NAMES) as they wait to adopt a child. You know the place where their child is now. Bind this precious child close to your breast and keep her/him secure. Let him/her not be afraid, but surround him/her with your loving Spirit.*
>
> *Be with his/her birth mother as she makes difficult decisions about adoption. We thank you for the new life she is sharing.*
>
> *We ask a special blessing upon (NAMES) as they wait to welcome their child home. Grant strength and courage to wait, for you know how they long to welcome their precious one home!*
>
> *Help them not to lose hope, as they wait and pray for their precious child. Be with them on this journey, and when they are together graft them into a strong and healthy family tree.*
>
> *All these things we pray in Jesus' name. Amen.*

56

Prayer for a Birth Mother

It takes a great deal of courage to give a child up for adoption. Sharing the precious life of a child with another family is a gift that is beyond all measure. Carrying a child, giving birth, and then letting go are profound acts of commitment to the dignity and worth of the whole human family.

Bless this birth mother, O God, who has carried and nurtured this child into birth. Comfort her as she releases this infant into the love and care of another family. Let the spiritual and loving bonds that were forged between birth mother and child remain, even as new bonds grow within a new forever family.

Bless her for her gift of life to this child and his/her new family. Sustain her in the days and years ahead as she remembers the child to whom she has given life. This time is a time both of tremendous joy and tremendous loss. Please comfort her.

Remind her, O God, that you promise to be with her child always, through growing years and into adulthood. Help her to know that she will always be an important piece of this child's life, even as she shares him/her with the family who will raise and also love this child forever.

Help her both to look back with thanksgiving for the life of this precious little one, and to look forward to the fullness of life that is ahead for them both in their separate yet always-joined ways. In your Holy Name we pray. Amen.

57

Prayer for Those with Mental Illness

The unknowns of mental illness are profound. Will this person respond to treatment? Will he/she recover? Will they be able to care for themselves when their family is gone? Will they be victims of crime, of cruelty, of shame, of sorrow? Who will love them? Who will make their heart sing?

> *Unsearchable God, who knows the minds and the reasoning of us all, have mercy on those suffering from mental illnesses and disorders. Lead them to compassionate healers and help-ful treatment. Surround them with encouragement; help them to love themselves as you love them and to know the joy of true friendship.*
>
> *Help us who love and care for them and about them not to despair, but to forge new paths of compromise that lead to a future and hope. When we ache for those who are afflicted, bring consolation that in you all people are whole. When we worry for them, send sojourners to surround them with dignity and purpose. When we weep for them, bring the comfort of assurance that you will never leave them or turn from them. We know, Comforting God, that there is nowhere, including the depths of depression, confusion, or delusion, that we can go from your sheltering presence.*
>
> *God of healing and hope, we pray for a day when all suffering and sorrowing will end. May that day come soon. We pray in your Holy Name. Amen.*

58

Prayer for a Child Who has been Abused

Prevent Child Abuse America, a national organization dedicated to protecting children, reminds us that child abuse and neglect occur in all segments of our society. For more information, visit the Web site of Prevent Child Abuse America at www.preventchildabuse.org or call them at 312-663-3520.

Loving Father and Mother God, let the tender mercy of your love enfold this, your precious child. Help him/her to recover from his/her physical wounds and begin the long, long journey to healing of mind and spirit. Help us make a safe place for him/her to go from here.

You understand the stressors of our lives — be with those who have hurt this child and help us to support them in finding ways to break the pattern of anguish and violence that has afflicted them. If it is found that this child is to be moved into a new home, let it be into a safe and supportive home where bonds of love and caring can begin to bring healing and hope to all.

We pray that you would help us work together to bring about a day when violence against all your precious children would cease. In your sacred name we pray, Amen.

59

Prayer for an Adult Who has been Abused

While certainly there are men who experience abuse at the hands of others, the majority of those who are abused in situations of domestic violence are women and children. The pronouns in this prayer reflect that reality and should be changed as is appropriate.

The National Domestic Violence Hotline is 1-800-799-7233.

Deal tenderly, O God, with this your precious one, who has been treated so unkindly by one who is close to her heart. Heal the wounds of her body and of her spirit. Speak words of kindness to her, and help her to hear them and to believe that such kindness is possible and true for her life. Teach her again to speak kindly to herself.

Bring hope, loving God, to the broken places in (NAME's) life, and help to find places where she (and her children) will be safe and can begin again. Let her healing over time bring newness of life — a way through the wilderness. Let healing streams of mercy flow where tears of pain run now.

Speak mercy, sheltering God, to one who finds herself in such a place of pain and sorrow. Grant her the strength to find a way through this ordeal and helpers to guide her into a place of safety and hope. Bless her and keep her in your loving care as she plants new seeds of wholeness in courage and strength. Let her lean upon your eternal and everlasting arms.

In Jesus' name we pray. Amen.

60

Prayer for Healing of the Earth

The health of our earth is critical to our personal and communal health. This prayer lifts up healing for God's creation, in which we are called to play a part.

God of all creation, we know that we cannot be whole unless we are able to live in harmony with the earth that nourishes and refreshes us. We pray that you would open our eyes to the personal and corporate ways we contribute to the earth's suffering.

Forgive our constant lusting after material goods, which consume earth's treasure and lay waste its fields when the possessions we have grow stale. Enliven our spirits, and help us to embrace lifestyles and choices that bring renewal to the earth's resources and living creatures.

Let us plant hope and tread lightly. Let us share and not hoard. Let us touch the earth gently, and let us mindfully recall daily the gifts and graciousness of the earth.

From brilliant birdsongs to fragrant flowers of the field, from refreshing breezes to resplendent harvest, we give thanks for the splendor and blessing of your sustaining creation. May we live in such a way that we become a blessing in return to all creation.

We lift our hearts in thanksgiving and gratitude for the fullness of life, shared by all living things on earth. We praise your goodness and your marvelous bounty, and ask that you help us be worthy of such a precious gift.

This we pray in your holy and everlasting name. Amen.

61

The Prayer of Our Savior (Paraphrase)

Sometimes hearing old words in new ways is a helpful way to pray. You might try saying the Prayer of Our Savior (the Lord's Prayer) very slowly and meditatively. It has quite a different effect on our hearts from saying the words in the way we usually say them in unison.

This paraphrase was written as a meditation on the Prayer of Our Savior, which is found in the sixth chapter of the Gospel of Matthew, and is one of the most profoundly beautiful prayers in a religious text. In it, Jesus changes the idea of God's persona from a vastly removed deity to a familiar, intimate, caring Presence.

> *Loving and everlasting Parent,*
> *who lives within our hearts, minds, and souls,*
> *and everywhere around us,*
> *hold us close to you, in mystery and holiness,*
> *as we glorify your sacred name.*
> *May your realm of justice and compassion*
> *come upon all the earth.*
> *May our lives reflect the integrity of your*
> *powerful, redeeming love.*
> *May all of us have enough of earth's bounty*
> *to live this day with thanksgiving, and without fear.*
> *Forgive us the many ways we hurt each other,*
> *and teach us new ways to forgive each other.*
> *When we are tempted by the world's power and riches,*
> *save us from ourselves, and make us truly your people.*

For all good comes from you,
*   and your ways transform and transcend our living,*
now and forever. Amen.

final word

Just a final note about these meditations and prayers. Please feel free to use them as you wish. Use the prayers verbatim, or adapt them for the situation in which a different prayer is needed. Use the meditations for personal reflection or as part of a devotional for a meeting or worship.

All of these prayers and meditations were written over the course of several years, while I was working in several different health-care and congregational settings. Healers must form theological worldviews from the vantage points of the settings in which they find themselves. All healers must ask their own questions about the nature of God, the reason(s) for suffering in the world, and how to find meaning in life and work.

Healers are all expected, however, to have some healing words for those who are hurting. God bless us all on our common and solitary journeys.

bibliography

Adams, Carol J. *The Sexual Politics of Meat: A Feminist-Vegetarian Critical Theory.* New York: Continuum, 1991.

Bender, Sue. *Everyday Sacred: A Woman's Journey Home.* San Francisco: Harper, 1995.

Bingham, June. *Courage to Change: An Introduction to the Life and Thought of Reinhold Niebuhr.* New York: Charles Scribner, 1961.

Carson, Verna Benner and Harold G. Koenig. *Parish Nursing: Stories of Service and Care.* Radnor, Pa.: Templeton Foundation Press, 2002.

Deshpande, Shashi. *Come Up and Be Dead.* 1983. Reprint, Bangalore, India: Dronequille, 2003.

——————. *That Long Silence.* New Delhi: Penguin Books India, 1988.

——————. *The Dark Holds No Terrors.* New Delhi: Penguin Books India, 1980.

Dossey, Larry. *Healing Words: The Power of Prayer and the Practice of Medicine.* San Francisco: HarperCollins, 1993.

_____. *Meaning & Medicine: Lessons from a Doctor's Tales of Breakthrough and Healing.* New York: Bantam, 1991.

Edelman, Marian Wright. *Guide My Feet: Prayers and Meditations on Loving and Working for Children.* Boston: Beacon Press, 1995.

Frost, Robert. *Complete Poems of Robert Frost.* New York: Holt, Rinehart and Winston, 1964.

Homan, Daniel, and Lonni Collins Pratt. *Radical Hospitality.* Brewster, Mass.: Paraclete Press, 2002.

Kushner, Lawrence. *Invisible Lines of Connection: Sacred Stories of the Ordinary.* Woodstock, Vt.: Jewish Lights Press, 1998.

Luks, Allan, with Peggy Payne. *The Healing Power of Doing Good: The Health and Spiritual Benefits of Helping Others.* New York: Fawcett Columbine, 1991.

Muller, Wayne. *Sabbath: Finding Rest, Renewal and Delight in Our Busy Lives.* New York: Bantam, 1999.

Sahgal, Nayantara. *Mistaken Identity.* 1988. Reprint, New Delhi: HarperCollins India, 2003.

Siegel, Bernie S. *How to Live Between Office Visits.* New York: HarperCollins, 1993.

_____. *Love, Medicine & Miracles.* New York: Harper & Row, 1986.

Warren, Elizabeth, and Amelia Warren Tyagi. *The Two-Income Trap: Why Middle-Class Mothers and Fathers Are Going Broke.* New York: Basic Books, 2003.

Wuellner, Flora Slossan. *Forgiveness: The Passionate Journey.* Nashville, Tenn.: Upper Room Books, 2001.

_____. *Prayer, Stress and Our Inner Wounds.* Nashville, Tenn.: Upper Room Books, 1985.

notes

MEDITATION 1

1. Larry Dossey, M.D., *Healing Words: The Power of Prayer and the Practice of Medicine* (San Francisco: HarperCollins, 1993), xv.
2. Ibid., 209.
3. Ibid.

MEDITATION 3

1. June Bingham, *Courage to Change: An Introduction to the Life and Thought of Reinhold Niebuhr* (New York: Charles Scribner, 1991), iii.
2. Ibid., 320.

MEDITATION 4

1. Allan Luks with Peggy Payne, *The Healing Power of Doing Good: The Health and Spiritual Benefits of Helping Others* (New York: Fawcett Columbine, 1991), 34-36.

2. Ibid., 12-16.

3. Ibid., 174-77.

MEDITATION 5

1. Sue Bender, *Everyday Sacred: A Woman's Journey Home* (San Francisco: Harper, 1995), 38.

2. Ibid., 96-97.

3. From the text of a personal letter to Sisters Madeleine Chollet, St. Pierre Cinquin, and Mary Agnes Boisson in Lyons, France, from Bishop Claude Marie Dubuis in San Antonio, Texas, 1869, which became the "founding letter" for their order in the United States and in Latin America. Source: Sisters of Charity of the Incarnate Word, San Antonio, *http://www.amormeus.org/*.

MEDITATION 7

1. Marian Wright Edelman, *Guide My Feet: Prayers and Meditations on Loving and Working for Children* (Boston: Beacon Press, 1995), 68.

MEDITATION 8

1. Rabbi Lawrence Kushner, *Invisible Lines of Connection: Sacred Stories of the Ordinary* (Woodstock, Vt: Jewish Lights Press, 1998), 40.

MEDITATION 10

1. Father Daniel Homan, OSB, and Lonni Collins Pratt, *Radical Hospitality* (Brewster, Mass.: Paraclete Press, 2002), 17-18.

MEDITATION 12

1. Verse one of "Once to Every Man and Nation," words by James R. Lowell, altered by W. Garrett Horder. *The Pilgrim Hymnal* (Boston: The Pilgrim Press, 1935), 326.

2. Ibid., verse five.

MEDITATION 13

1. Unpublished personal records of Sister Bena Fuchs, 1914, Deaconess Hospital Archives, St. Louis, Missouri.

MEDITATION 14

1. As quoted by Leon Eden in *Henry James: The Master* (Philadelphia: J. B. Lippincott, 1972), 519. Original letter to Clare Sheridan is part of the Berg Collection, 1867-1917, Henry James Papers, The New York Public Library.

MEDITATION 15

1. Verses three and four of "O Grant Us, God, A Little Space" by John Ellerton, from Thomas Este's *Whole Book of Psalmes* (1592).
2. Ibid., verse five.

MEDITATION 19

1. "Don't Worry, Be Healthy?" *Mirabella,* January/February 1997, vol. 8, no. 1, 50-55.

MEDITATION 20

1. "Arrest Declining Sex Ratio," *The Hindu,* 11 July 2004.
2. Shashi Deshpande, *Come Up and Be Dead* (1983; Bangalore, India: Dronequille, 2003), 105.
3. Nayantara Sahgal, *Mistaken Identity* (1988; reprint, New Delhi: HarperCollins India 2003), 63-64.
4. Shirley Geok-Lin Lim, interview by Bill Moyers, in *Fooling with Words: A Celebration of Poets and their Craft* (New York: Perennial, 2001), 134-36. Poem used with permission of the author.
5. "Abandoned Baby Finds a Home," *Deccan Herald,* 30 July 2004.

MEDITATION 21

1. "Antidepressant Use Growing in Children," *The New York Times,* 2 April 2004.

2. "New Lessons for College Students: Lighten Up," *The New York Times*, 6 April 2004.

3. Wayne Muller, *Sabbath: Finding Rest, Renewal, and Delight in Our Busy Lives* (New York: Bantam, 1999), 8-9.

PRAYER 50

1. Elizabeth Warren and Amelia Warren Tyagi, *The Two-Income Trap: Why Middle-Class Mothers and Fathers Are Going Broke* (New York: Basic Books, 2003), 6.

OTHER BOOKS FROM THE PILGRIM PRESS

THE ESSENTIAL PARISH NURSE
ABCs for Congregational Health Ministry
Deborah Patterson

This practical and useful resource is designed for churches that want to develop a parish nurse program. Covering a broad range, it discusses the need for such ministry, a brief history of parish nursing, the role of the parish nurse, and other details of interest to those wishing to establish such a ministry.

ISBN 0-8298-1571-6
Paper, 160 pages
$18.00

THE HEALING CHURCH
Practical Programs for Health Ministries
Abigail Rian Evans

What role can churches and religious organizations play in health care today? Abigail Rian Evans answers this question and others in this valuable guide to practical programs for health ministries. It includes a vast list of existing ministries that can be used as models.

ISBN 0-8298-1309-8
Paper, 260 pages
$24.00

REDEEMING MARKETPLACE MEDICINE
A Theology of Health Care
Abigail Rian Evans

Evans asserts that corporate-based managed care places profits over patient care. She further points out that medical experts have reduced health care to medical treatment under arrangements with health insurance plans and health maintenance organizations. Providing an engaging Christian theology, Evans proposes a broader health care model.

ISBN 0-8298-1310-1
Paper, 208 pages
$17.00

SOUL CALLING
Breathing Life into a Life of Service
Julie Ruth Harley

Harley identifies difficulties presented by ministries that create stumbling blocks to spiritual growth. Writing in a personal meditative tone, Harley presents spiritually nourishing activities that will enable those in service ministries to develop their spiritual discipline — and deepen the sense of meaning in their lives and ministries.

ISBN 0-8298-1278-4
Paper, 144 pages
$16.00

HEALTH AS LIBERATION
Medicine, Theology and the Quest for Justice
Alastair V. Campbell

In this lucid and moving analysis of what constitutes a theologically grounded understanding of authentic health care, ethicist Campbell relates the cases of those not often heard — those vulnerable patients in hospital wards. He demonstrates convincingly why all of us — both inside and outside of Washington — need to listen.

ISBN 0-8298-1022-6
Cloth, 112 pages
$15.00

MEDICINE AS MINISTRY
Reflections on Suffering, Ethics and Hope
Margaret E. Mohrmann, M.D.

How does one begin to reconcile faith in a merciful God with the crushing reality of human suffering? Over twenty years, Mohrmann has sought to heal children racked by disease and dysfunction, helping many to recover — and watching some die. This book is her moving story of the implications of a theological understanding of health, illness, and hope.

ISBN 0-8298-1073-0
Paper, 120 pages
$13.00

PAIN SEEKING UNDERSTANDING
Suffering, Medicine, and Faith
Margaret E. Mohrmann and Mark J. Hanson, editors

This resource examines how believers and nonbelievers alike wrestle with questions of faith when confronted with pain and suffering that medicine alone cannot treat. Fellow experts in the fields of medicine, ethics, theology, and pastoral care help to weave the complex story of faith and science.

ISBN 0-8298-1354-3
Paper, 224 pages
$2.30 net

TO ORDER THESE OR ANY OTHER BOOKS FROM THE PILGRIM PRESS CALL OR WRITE TO:

The Pilgrim Press
700 Prospect Avenue East
Cleveland, Ohio 44115-1100

Phone orders: **1-800-537-3394** or Fax orders: **216-736-2206**
Please include shipping charges of $4.00 for the first book and $0.75 for each additional book.
Or order from our Web sites at *www.pilgrimpress.com* and *www.ucpress.com*.

Prices subject to change without notice.